"Colleen Carney and Rachel Manber clearly understand the broad domain of insomnia and the suffering it causes. Their book reflects the authors' deep knowledge of sleep medicine and their experience treating hundreds of insomnia sufferers. It will no doubt help millions more as it clearly explains not only what to do, but also why. I sincerely wish *Quiet Your Mind and Get to Sleep* had been available sooner."

> —William C. Dement, MD, Ph.D., professor of psychiatry and sleep medicine at Stanford University School of Medicine and author of *The Promise of Sleep*

"People with insomnia have been told for years that insomnia will go away if they get treatment for depression, anxiety, or pain, and this often does not happen. What is needed is a straightforward practical guide to solving their sleep issues, and these two leading experts in comorbid insomnias deliver. *Quiet Your Mind and Get to Sleep* is sensitive to the types of challenges faced by people with complicated health issues while taking a no-nonsense approach to eliminating the factors known to perpetuate sleep problems. The chapters and worksheets are interactive—it is like having access to your own therapist. This is a timely and truly essential book for anyone who suffers from insomnia and those who love them."

> —Jack D. Edinger, Ph.D., CBSM, clinical professor in the department of psychiatry and behavioral sciences at Duke University Medical Center and senior psychologist at Durham VA Medical Center

"Carney and Manber have written an incredibly useful guide book for individuals with insomnia, especially insomnia that occurs with depression, pain, and anxiety. It is full of practical strategies and tools for self-care, clearly explained, with great examples from real insomnia sufferers. *Quiet Your Mind and Get to Sleep* walks you through all the key elements of behavioral treatment that you would get from a sleep specialist. I will definitely recommend it to my patients with insomnia."

> —Daniel J. Buysse, MD, professor of psychiatry and clinical and translational science at the University of Pittsburgh School of Medicine

D1120447

"Dr. Rachel Manber's new book *Quiet Your Mind and Get to Sleep* is the next best thing one can do after travelling to Stanford University to receive her insomnia therapy. She is a one of the world's experts in insomnia research and a master of creating personalized, creative, and effective treatment plans for insomnia. Her methods go above and beyond the usual don't read in bed techniques and translate into results. This book is important because education is a key component to treating insomnia."

> —Meredith Broderick, MD
> Medical Director of the Sleep Center at Minor and James Medical
> A Swedish Health Partner

"What can compare in beneficent impact on our minds and moods with a good night's sleep? In *Quiet Your Mind and Get to Sleep*, Carney and Manber do a masterful job of digesting the latest science for lay readers interested in improving their sleep. A unique feature of this work is its thorough treatment of the complicating factors of mood disturbances and chronic pain. This book stakes out an important place in sleep and health literature."

> —Steven H. Woodward, Ph.D., director of the Sleep Research Laboratory,
> National Center for PTSD

quiet your mind & get to sleep

solutions to insomnia
for those with depression,
anxiety, or chronic pain

COLLEEN E. CARNEY, PH.D.
RACHEL MANBER, PH.D.

New Harbinger Publications, Inc.

Publisher's Note

Care has been taken to confirm the accuracy of the information presented and to describe generally accepted practices. However, the authors, editors, and publisher are not responsible for errors or omissions or for any consequences from application of the information in this book and make no warranty, express or implied, with respect to the contents of the publication.

The authors, editors, and publisher have exerted every effort to ensure that any drug selection and dosage set forth in this text are in accordance with current recommendations and practice at the time of publication. However, in view of ongoing research, changes in government regulations, and the constant flow of information relating to drug therapy and drug reactions, the reader is urged to check the package insert for each drug for any change in indications and dosage and for added warnings and precautions. This is particularly important when the recommended agent is a new or infrequently employed drug.

Some drugs and medical devices presented in this publication may have Food and Drug Administration (FDA) clearance for limited use in restricted research settings. It is the responsibility of the health care provider to ascertain the FDA status of each drug or device planned for use in their clinical practice.

NEW HARBINGER PUBLICATIONS is a registered trademark of New Harbinger Publications, Inc.

Distributed in Canada by Raincoast Books

Copyright © 2009 by Colleen E. Carney and Rachel Manber
New Harbinger Publications, Inc.
5720 Shattuck Avenue
Oakland, CA 94609
www.newharbinger.com

Cover design by Amy Shoup; Text design by Tracy Carlson; Acquired by Jess O'Brien; Edited by Nelda Street

Library of Congress Cataloging in Publication Data

Carney, Colleen.
   Quiet your mind and get to sleep : solutions to insomnia for those with depression, anxiety, or chronic pain / Colleen E. Carney and Rachel Manber.
       p. cm.
   Includes bibliographical references and index.
   ISBN-13: 978-1-57224-627-0 (pbk. : alk. paper)
   ISBN-10: 1-57224-627-8 (pbk. : alk. paper) 1. Insomnia--Popular works. 2. Depression--Complications--Popular works. 3. Anxiety--Complications--Popular works. 4. Chronic pain--Complications--Popular works. I. Manber, Rachel. II. Title.
   RC548.C367 2009
   616.8'4982--dc22   2009038434

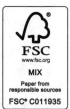

Printed in the United States of America

25   24   23

20   19   18

For Shannon and Sydney
—C.E.C.

For Udi, Tali, and Shelly
—R.M.

contents

foreword

I heard a voice cry, "Sleep no more!
Macbeth does murder sleep,"—the innocent sleep;
Sleep that knits up the ravell'd sleave of care,
The death of each day's life, sore labour's bath,
Balm of hurt minds, great nature's second course,
Chief nourisher in life's feast.

—Shakespeare, *Macbeth*

The importance of sleep has been recognized for centuries. Sleep was understood by Shakespeare to heal emotional and cognitive distress ("knits up the ravell'd sleave of care," "balm of hurt minds") as well as physical aches and pains ("sore labour's bath"). Today's researchers have confirmed the central role that sleep plays in almost every aspect of human life, including regulating emotion; reducing stress, worry, and irritability; consolidating memories; improving cognitive performance; reducing pain; strengthening the immune system; and reducing daytime fatigue and sleepiness. In today's twenty-four-hour, seven-day-a-week world, sleep disturbance is a common problem. For many people, this leads to chronic insomnia. Because of the central role that sleep has in emotional, cognitive, and physical functioning, problems in these other areas may develop or be made worse when sleep is disturbed.

The authors of this workbook, Drs. Colleen Carney and Rachel Manber, are experienced sleep clinicians who are among the world's leading researchers examining the treatment of insomnia in people who have additional emotional, cognitive, or physical problems. This workbook is unique among books available in providing the knowledge and skills to treat insomnia in ways that promise to produce the full range of benefits to those with depression or pain or other problems along with insomnia.

Is there evidence that treating sleep will improve other problems such depression or pain? The answer is a resounding yes, and Drs. Carney and Manber have published the watershed studies that have provided that evidence. Their book is a comprehensive, integrative approach to cognitive behavioral therapy for insomnia. One of its best features is the many self-assessments to guide the reader in applying the treatment recommendations. This reflects an active learning perspective that will help the reader truly master the skills and strategies.

It is ironic that society's increasing recognition of the importance of sleep may make the treatment of insomnia more difficult. As is made clear in the workbook, people with sleep disturbances often have unrealistic expectations about sleep and exaggerated concerns about the effects of even a single night of poor sleep. A central aspect of the workbook is to teach skills to help identify expectations that are not realistic and to help substitute alternative statements and actions. Those with insomnia put pressure on themselves to sleep better. As the workbook chapters point out, this can often lead to behaviors that make better sleep less likely.

Instead, we need to recognize that sleep is indeed important, as Shakespeare recognized, but that sleep cannot be forced to occur. The solution is to engage knowledge and skills that allow for sleep. The authors have struck just the right balance between the importance of sleep and the methods for improving sleep in this outstanding workbook.

—Richard R. Bootzin, Ph.D.
   professor and director, Insomnia Program
   Departments of Psychology and Psychiatry
   University of Arizona
   Tucson, Arizona

introduction

Modern society often dictates long hours, packed schedules, and less time to sleep and to unwind. To "stay ahead" in their work lives, North Americans don't take as many vacations as they used to, which is unfortunate, because in a fast-paced and busy life, taking time to unwind and recharge your battery is more important than ever. So it's understandable that insomnia is the number-one health problem in Western societies (Canals et al. 1997). Sleep requires disengaging from the bustling environment around us, and stress interferes with this process. Stress can come in many forms, possibly arising in the context of a major life event, such as taking a new job, becoming a parent, or ending a relationship. It's no surprise that these stressful situations are often associated with difficulty sleeping. In addition, the experience of disturbed sleep is itself a source of stress that tends to further prolong the problem. That is, when you have difficulty sleeping, you begin to worry about being able to sleep at night and being able to function the next day, and that worry makes it more difficult to sleep. When sleep difficulties persist and lead to daytime problems, such as irritability, depressed mood, difficulty concentrating, or fatigue, the sleep problem often calls for a medical diagnosis of insomnia.

More often than not, insomnia occurs along with other health problems, most commonly depression, anxiety, and chronic pain conditions. Each of these three problems can cause you considerable personal suffering, not to mention the cost of medications and visits to the doctor's office. The suffering and societal costs are even higher when you have insomnia along with depression, anxiety, or chronic pain, a kind of insomnia called *comorbid* insomnia. Yet until recently, doctors didn't usually treat comorbid insomnia, because they assumed that it was merely a symptom of the other health problem and would go away when the other problem was treated. However, untreated comorbid insomnia often doesn't get better even after the other condition is adequately treated (Carney et al. 2007), and untreated insomnia can make the other condition worse or interfere with its treatment (Carney et al. 2007; Buysse et al. 1999). For example, when treated for their coexisting depression, people with insomnia don't improve as much as those without sleep difficulties (Buysse et al. 1999). For reasons like this, the National Institutes of Health (NIH), the leading health-research funding agency in the United States, recently released a statement that urges doctors to treat the insomnia that occurs along with another conditions (National Institutes of Health 2005).

In that vein, this book describes an effective insomnia treatment called *cognitive behavioral therapy* (CBT). Some readers might be familiar with CBT for other mental disorders, such as depression, anxiety disorders, and eating disorders. They all share common principles but use some problem-specific techniques. CBT for insomnia has been tested in many studies, and the results show that CBT is an effective treatment, just as effective as taking sleep medications (Smith et al. 2002). Most important, when people are followed for a period after the end of treatment, the sleep improvements seen at the end of treatment last longest in those treated with CBT (Edinger et al. 2001; Morin et al. 1999). We highlight this information because it's very relevant to the insomnia that occurs in the context of another medical or mental condition, which is our focus. In people who have both insomnia and depression:

- Whether your treatment involves antidepressant medication or psychotherapy, insomnia remains a significant issue for about half of those who recover from depression (Carney et al. 2007).

- Having insomnia increases your risk of developing depression in the future (Ford and Kamerow 1989).

Taking these facts together, we can conclude that an insomnia treatment with longer-lasting effects will also have a more favorable effect on depression.

The approach we describe in this book provides practical advice in enough detail to allow you to apply it to your situation. Because we have written this CBT self-help workbook for people who have insomnia along with another condition, we provide specific suggestions for issues related to experiencing insomnia along with another health problem. Let's continue with our example of insomnia occurring with depression. Some of the CBT recommendations aren't easy to follow and might seem particularly difficult to those who also have depression. For instance, CBT recommends that people get out of bed shortly after waking up in the morning. This recommendation is challenging for many people with depression, because they often find it difficult to get started in the morning. Therefore we give specific suggestions on how to overcome this challenge. We also discuss tools to manage the high levels of anxiety that are common to many people with depression, anxiety, and pain. We also provide methods for dealing with common daytime consequences of poor sleep, such as low energy, trouble concentrating, and irritable mood. Again, this is very important in the context of depression, because low energy, poor concentration, and irritability are also symptoms of depression. Our approach also emphasizes the importance of the mind in insomnia and offers many practical suggestions for dealing with an overactive mind or anxiety-provoking thoughts. People with insomnia often complain of having a "noisy mind" at night, particularly those who are more anxious than average or describe themselves as "perfectionists." We recognize that each person is unique and faces different challenges when being treated for insomnia, and we hope you'll find that this approach fits your particular set of challenges.

Quiet Your Mind and Get to Sleep provides strategies to overcome the insomnia that occurs with other conditions. Each chapter focuses on providing sleep-related information, self-tests, and simple worksheets to help you enact changes in thoughts or behaviors known to perpetuate insomnia. Each treatment recommendation is made in the context of understanding what's going on in the accompanying disorder. As such, this book is for anyone who has ever struggled with insomnia and for those who love them.

You may be wondering whether you can use this book if you're taking medication, and the short answer is yes. This approach is effective even when you're taking medication for sleep, pain, anxiety, or depression. You may have read that some antidepressant medications cause insomnia as a side effect. This may happen with certain antidepressant medications, but it's not very common. You may wonder whether you should discontinue antidepressant medications just in case they're causing the insomnia. If insomnia emerges as a side effect of an antidepressant medication and it doesn't go away in a few weeks, your prescribing physician will likely offer an alternative antidepressant medication because people react differently to these medications. Don't stop taking prescribed medications without first consulting with the physician who prescribed them. Stopping medications abruptly and without guidance can be very uncomfortable and sometimes dangerous. Stopping sleep medications can result in *rebound insomnia*, which is caused by stopping the medication and doesn't necessarily reflect your underlying sleep patterns. If you stopped taking prescribed medication for depression or anxiety, this condition could worsen, making it difficult for you to follow the sleep treatment we offer. Besides, even if you believe that a medication has a negative impact on your sleep quality, it's unlikely that your insomnia would resolve the moment you stopped taking it. You can discuss with your physician any concerns you might have about your medications. If you have pain, anxiety, or depression, continue to get treatment for these conditions. In all likelihood, it will be easier for you to follow the instructions for the insomnia treatment described in this book when your pain, depression, or anxiety is under control.

Our approach doesn't require that you stop whatever therapy you're currently receiving. In fact, we hope that if you have a coexisting condition, you're getting treatment and your treatment provider is available to assist you with using the strategies in this book. We believe that the best approach to treating insomnia in the context of another condition is to treat both conditions. Making health-related changes can be quite demanding, and how you decide to make such changes is a personal choice. While we've written the sleep strategies so that you can use them on your own, you may wish to enlist the help of a sleep specialist in your area. By providing information about sleep and helpful exercises, this book will offer you an opportunity to take control of your insomnia. We hope you'll discover that making small changes in the way you approach sleep will give you the sleep you dream about!

the scope of the insomnia problem

Retired CEO Garry came to the sleep clinic because he was having trouble falling asleep. He would toss and turn for an hour or two before finally being able to fall asleep, a problem that began when he was in college. He'd tried a variety of different sleeping pills over the years but continued to have trouble sleeping. In recent years, he'd taken to drinking a martini every evening to help him "unwind." He usually began feeling sleepy by around 11:00 p.m., which was when he headed upstairs to bed. However, as soon as he got into bed, he felt wide awake. He tossed and turned, and after a while thought, "Ugh, it's happening again; how long can this go on?" After enduring almost an hour of frustration about being unable to fall asleep, he would take a sleeping pill or drink more alcohol, and finally fall asleep between 12:30 and 1:00 a.m. Once asleep, he slept fine but would wake up and get out of bed between 7:00 and 8:00 a.m., feeling as if his head were "clogged up." This had gone on several times a week for much of his adult life. Having had anxiety problems for as long as he could remember, Garry believed that his insomnia and anxiety were linked. He recalled that the insomnia first began in college, when he experienced anxiety before taking examinations.

As we talked about his anxiety, he realized that he became worried in a variety of situations. He also worried that his insomnia would make him susceptible to a serious illness.

A senior in college, Frank began waking up in the middle of the night last winter, and would then be awake for hours. At first, this wasn't much of a problem, because he could take an afternoon nap and feel better for the rest of the day. Lately he found that despite feeling very tired, he couldn't sleep when he lay down for a nap. He started feeling down and was no longer excited about things he used to enjoy, such as jogging, playing Frisbee, and doing his schoolwork. Feeling bad about himself, he withdrew from his friends and began skipping classes. Sometimes he slept in and showed up late to classes. He even had to ask for extensions for some of his course work. He went to see a doctor at the student health clinic and was prescribed antidepressant medication. When the doctor asked him if he had ever been depressed before, Frank realized that he probably had been depressed in high school too. The antidepressant medication helped his mood significantly, but his insomnia continued. He became quite concerned that unless he started sleeping better, the depression would return. He believed that getting his sleep pattern back on track was the key to graduating.

A schoolteacher, Barbara had experienced problems falling asleep and waking up multiple times in the middle of the night. She was diagnosed with fibromyalgia several years ago, and still suffered with it. Her pain and fatigue fluctuated in severity, but even when these symptoms were under control, she continued to have problems sleeping. She tended to take over an hour to fall asleep and wake up two hours later with difficulty returning to sleep. After a few bad nights, her pain would increase. She became very frustrated because each of the sleeping medications that initially had been effective stopped working. In an attempt to get more sleep, she started going to bed earlier than usual and resting in the morning hours, but nothing seemed to help.

The three people in these case scenarios had something in common: they all experienced insomnia along with another health-related condition. Garry suffered from anxiety, Frank had a history of depression, and Barbara struggled with chronic pain. This chapter will provide you with a description of insomnia as well as the disorders that commonly co-occur with insomnia, including depression, anxiety, and chronic pain. We'll outline the common symptoms of these disorders and discuss how insomnia impacts these conditions when they coexist with insomnia.

what is insomnia?

What problems in the people you just read about (whose names have been changed to protect their privacy) characterize them as having insomnia? We all experience sleep disruption from time to time, but when should we seek treatment? Usually, a person seeks treatment when the problem becomes persistent and has a significant impact on daytime functioning, which is how doctors distinguish between having difficulty sleeping and having an actual insomnia-disorder diagnosis. Generally, *insomnia* is disturbed sleep that's persistent (lasts more than a month) and causes other problems too. Other problems can include fatigue, mental "cloudiness," or mood problems, or it could mean that the sleep problem causes distress or interferes with usual activities. An example of a sleep problem interfering with activities is if you cancel appointments or call in sick for work because of poor sleep on the previous night. Other problems also include worsening of the symptoms of another condition, such as pain, anxiety, or depression; for example, Barbara, who has fibromyalgia, noticed that her pain tended to worsen after several nights of poor sleep.

More formally, doctors and other health providers diagnose insomnia, depression, and anxiety disorders based on a standardized diagnostic manual published by the American Psychiatric Association (APA). This manual, called the *Diagnostic and Statistical Manual of Mental Disorders* (*DSM*), was written based on input from experts in the mental health field from around the world. This panel of experts examined published research and conducted new studies. Based on this information the panel established diagnostic criteria for many disorders, including insomnia, mood, and anxiety disorders. The fourth edition of the *DSM* has a set of criteria for different types of insomnia disorders, including situations in which the insomnia meets one of the following conditions (APA 2000):

- Insomnia is the primary clinical complaint (primary insomnia).

- Insomnia occurs exclusively during a medical illness (insomnia related to a medical disorder).

- Insomnia occurs exclusively with a mental health condition (insomnia related to a mental disorder).

To be diagnosed with any type of insomnia disorder, both the nighttime and daytime criteria need to be met for at least one month. The nighttime criterion is the presence of difficulty falling or staying asleep, or feeling unrested in the morning. The daytime criterion is the presence of distress or concern about sleep, or other consequences of poor sleep. As noted previously, some of the consequences of poor sleep include fatigue; irritated, anxious, or depressed mood; achiness; difficulty concentrating; and finding it hard to do things at work, home, or school. Other sleep disorders, such as sleep apnea, which we'll describe in chapter 2, can have similar symptoms to insomnia, such as disturbed sleep, fatigue, and low energy. Therefore, another criterion for the diagnosis of insomnia is that the symptoms are not better accounted for by another sleep disorder. In other words, it must be insomnia rather than another sleep disorder that's producing the symptoms. If you're unsure whether or not you have another sleep disorder, please read the section "Could You Have Another Sleep Disorder?" in the next chapter.

insomnia is more common than you think

When an insomnia disorder is present for six months or more, it's called *chronic insomnia*. Most people who go to a sleep specialist to treat their insomnia have suffered symptoms for at least six months. Chronic insomnia is a problem for approximately one in ten adults (Ohayon 2002), which is a staggering number. Even more staggering is that the rate of sleep disturbance doubles in those over sixty-five years old (Foley et al. 1995). Because almost all stress-related conditions involve disturbed sleep, it's not surprising that the insomnia that occurs with another disorder is the most common type of insomnia among people with sleep problems. In fact, the number of sleep problems that occur with another condition is twice as high as the number of sleep problems that occur in the absence of another condition (Buysse et al. 1994). Insomnia can cause considerable personal suffering, as well as more frequent visits to the doctor and missed workdays. Whereas the costs and suffering associated with disorders such as depression, anxiety, and pain are substantial, they're particularly noteworthy among those who also have insomnia.

As discussed in the introduction, in the past it was assumed that when insomnia occurred with another medical or psychiatric disorder, the insomnia was simply a symptom of the other disorder. The assumption was that the insomnia would get better when the medical or psychiatric condition was adequately treated. We now know that this is not always true. Insomnia often doesn't get better when the accompanying condition is treated. More often, the insomnia merits separate attention and focused treatment. While it's true that depression, anxiety, and pain can, in some cases, cause sleep difficulties, with time the sleep difficulties can worsen and take on a life of their own. In other words, over time the sleep difficulties develop into an insomnia disorder. Often the insomnia persists even after the condition that originally caused it improves, which was the case for Frank; his depression resolved with antidepressant medication, but his sleep problem remained.

how do you know if you have depression or anxiety?

Having chronic pain is self-evident and probably needs no additional definition. Most people aren't surprised to learn that they have chronic pain; they simply feel it and are aware that it's an issue. When you have pain, you can easily track how it changes over time. In contrast, depression and anxiety disorders are sometimes more subtle. You may have a depressive or anxiety disorder without being aware of it. Or perhaps you know you have the disorder but you've had it for so long that you "forget" that it could be any different. Even if you've already been diagnosed with an anxiety or depressive disorder, you might benefit from gaining a better understanding of the criteria used to diagnose these disorders and from having a way to track their severity over time. So before proceeding, let's define specific depressive and anxiety disorders. While this information can't replace professional evaluation, it may help you decide whether you need to consult a health provider.

Indications of Possible Mood Disorders

Mood disorders are usually characterized by pervasive down, dejected mood episodes, commonly called *depression*; pervasive elevated, euphoric mood episodes, commonly called *mania* or *hypomania*; or both. We'll present signs for each type of mood disorder next.

depression

Here are some common signs of depression:

- You feel sad, empty, down, agitated, or angry more often than not.

- You have difficulty enjoying the things you normally like to do.

- You have trouble getting interested in things or have persistent trouble with motivation.

If you've had any of these problems more days than not for at least two or more weeks, get evaluated for depression. Most important, if you're having thoughts or images about harming yourself—for example, thinking "My family would be better off if I were dead" or picturing yourself driving off the road—don't dismiss them; seek a professional evaluation immediately. It's important to seek help in this situation in order to protect yourself from harm. Following are some other signs of depression:

- You've been withdrawing from the people you normally enjoy being around.

- On most days, you feel tired, have low energy, and drag through the day much of the time.

- You have insomnia (trouble falling or staying asleep, or waking too early in the morning) or the opposite problem: sleeping *too much*.

- You feel bad about yourself, struggle with poor self-esteem, or have self-critical thoughts more often than usual, or judge yourself as worthless.

- You struggle with guilty thoughts or thoughts related to feeling punished in some way.

- You've had an increase or decrease in appetite or weight (without consciously trying to lose weight).

- You or others notice that you either move or talk unusually slowly, or move or talk unusually fast.

- You have more difficulty making decisions than usual.

- You have greater difficulty concentrating or remembering things than usual.

bipolar disorder

Sometimes depression can alternate with what can be described as an *overly* excited, hyperactive, or agitated mood. We say "overly" excited because when you're in this mood state, others might comment that you're moving much more quickly than normal or talking faster than usual, or that you're very distractible. Having this hyperactive mood for a week or more might be a sign of what we call a *manic* or *hypomanic* state. Other signs of a manic state include:

- A decreased need to sleep, which differs from insomnia in that you may feel as though you don't *need* to sleep or that you require very little sleep (for example, needing less than four hours, when normally you would sleep substantially longer)

- Unusually high self-esteem or having an unrealistic sense that you can do anything (for example, you suddenly devote all your time to composing a symphony even though you have no musical training or ability)

- A racing or continuous stream of thoughts

- Engaging in an excessive amount of activities or doing things to excess

- Engaging in uncharacteristically reckless behavior, including lavish spending sprees, sexual promiscuity, risky business ventures, or illegal activity

- The mood described above results in your being admitted to a hospital or experiencing some other negative consequence (for example, being arrested)

As you may be able to discern from the previous description, several symptoms pose potential danger during a manic state. The presence of a manic or hypomanic state characterizes the diagnosis of *bipolar disorder* (formerly *manic-depressive disorder*) or a similar condition called *cyclothymia*. These conditions involve an alternation between overly excited and depressed mood states, which can greatly disrupt the lives of people suffering from this disorder, as well as those of their families. The treatment of depression in someone who has experienced a manic episode in the past differs from that of someone who has never had such an experience. If you recognize several of the previously described signs, seek medical advice.

Indications of Possible Anxiety Disorders Involving Insomnia

In addition to depressive disorders, anxiety disorders also commonly occur with insomnia. Following are examples of such disorders.

chronic worry

A certain level of worry can be constructive; for example, worrying about the success of an upcoming event propels us to prepare for it, and worrying about a problem makes us seek solutions. However, sometimes we worry about things that are out of our control, or we worry too much and freeze rather than use the worry to solve a problem, which was the case with Garry. He found himself worrying so much that he seemed to worry about everything, to the point where the worries seemed unmanageable. Excessive worry can be a sign of *generalized anxiety disorder* (GAD), which is characterized by the following symptoms:

- The worry is excessive, meaning that it occupies a substantial amount of time and may be out of proportion relative to other people's response to the same situation.

- The worry is uncontrollable to a certain degree; for example, you understand that the worry is excessive but nevertheless find it difficult to stop worrying.

- The worries aren't limited to just one or two topics; for example, you may worry about coping during the day after a poor night's sleep. However, if this is the *only* thing you're excessively worried about, you don't have this symptom.

- The worry is associated with physical symptoms, such as muscle tension, stomach upset, irritable mood, feeling "keyed up" or agitated, or having problems concentrating.

If you have some of these symptoms most days for at least six months, consult a mental health professional.

panic attacks

Some people experience panic attacks, characterized by intense anxiety that's distinct from anxious mood or mild chronic anxiety. Sometimes panic attacks arise in people with chronic levels of anxiety but not always. The word "attack" means that the experience is sudden, often out of the blue. Panic attacks are a sudden rush of symptoms that often resolve almost as quickly as they began. From start to finish, panic attacks usually last about ten minutes. During a panic attack, typically several of the following symptoms occur:

- Pounding heart, palpitations, rapid heart rate, or chest pain or discomfort

- Sweating, trembling, or shaking

- Shortness of breath, or sensations of choking or smothering

- Nausea or stomach upset

- Dizziness, faintness, or light-headedness

- Feeling as if things aren't "real"

- Feeling as if you're detached from yourself (for example, some people describe feeling as if they're floating outside the body)

- Experiencing fears of losing control or "going crazy," or fears that you might die during the event

- Numbness or tingling sensations, chills, or hot flashes

Many people may experience an isolated panic attack or two in a lifetime, and this, in itself, is not a diagnosable disorder. There are, however, circumstances in which a panic attack is a symptom of an anxiety disorder, called *panic disorder*, which is a condition diagnosed in people who have had at least one panic attack and persistently (for example, for at least one month) fear having another attack, or are concerned about the implications of the attacks. This may mean that the person fears that the panic signifies something more serious, such as a heart attack. Because of symptoms such as heart palpitations and shortness of breath, it's not uncommon for people enduring a panic attack to go to the emergency room fearing that they're having a heart attack. Sometimes the main fear is about losing control. Some people with panic disorder avoid situations they fear would trigger a panic attack or would be particularly embarrassing should an attack occur. People with panic disorder may avoid situations in which they think it might be difficult to escape.

People with panic disorder are sometimes woken from sleep by a panic attack, which is called a *nocturnal panic attack*. Some experience only nocturnal panic; that is, they don't regularly have daytime panic attacks. In addition to disturbing sleep, nocturnal panic can increase anxiety about sleeping, leading to fear of going to sleep.

post-traumatic stress disorder

Sometimes people can develop anxiety problems after experiencing a serious trauma, a condition known as *post-traumatic stress disorder* (PTSD). Most often these are situations in which a person was seriously injured or could have been killed, but it can also happen when a person witnesses someone else's serious injury or death. Examples of trauma include crimes such as rape, natural disasters such as tornadoes, or involvement in combat or vehicular accidents. But having experienced a trauma is not enough to warrant a diagnosis. There are several other components of a PTSD diagnosis; for example, there's often unwanted reexperiencing of that traumatic event. Reexperiencing can occur in any of the following ways:

- Repeated unwanted memories of the traumatic event

- "Flashbacks," or a sense of reliving the event

- Recurrent nightmares about the event

- Intense fear or emotional distress when in the presence of reminders of the event

In addition, the event is so traumatic that it produces arousal symptoms, such as:

- Insomnia

- Irritability or angry outbursts

- Difficulties concentrating

- Always feeling "on guard" against something "bad" happening

- Having an overly sensitive startle response (for instance, if someone sneaked up on you, you'd be much more startled than someone without PTSD)

If you suffer from PTSD, you may tend to avoid situations that remind you of the trauma, which includes avoiding people, places, thoughts, or activities that could cause you to think about the trauma. People with PTSD may also forget aspects of the trauma. You may begin to feel numb, have difficulty experiencing the full range of human emotion, and have difficulty interacting with people. Instead, your interactions may seem unreal or detached in some way. It's not uncommon for people with PSTD to believe they'll have a shortened life.

obsessive-compulsive disorder

Obsessive-compulsive disorder (OCD) is characterized by intrusive unwanted, anxiety-provoking thoughts or images, followed by a compulsive strategy to get rid of them. Such a strategy typically involves rituals such as repeated counting, washing, or checking (for example, checking whether locks are actually locked or whether appliances are turned off). People who suffer from this condition recognize that the obsessions and compulsive behavior are irrational or excessive, but feel helpless to resist it, which is a particularly frustrating experience for someone with OCD. OCD can be a debilitating condition that impacts work productivity and relationships. However, it rarely interferes with sleep unless the rituals occur at night; for example, being compelled over and over to check and recheck that all the doors are locked before going to sleep will interfere with falling asleep at night.

social phobia

Social phobia is a diagnosis characterized by a persistent and pronounced fear of social situations, the most fear-provoking of which tend to be those where your performance (social or otherwise) could be judged by others, or new or unfamiliar people are involved. The fear is best described as one of embarrassment, which could mean that you're concerned that you'll show anxiety symptoms in public or be humiliated in some way. People with social phobia tend to avoid social interactions as much as possible, and in cases where they can't avoid a social setting, they experience intense anxiety and possibly even a panic attack (see previous description of panic attacks). The cycle of anticipatory anxiety, avoidance of social or performance situations, and the intensity of anxiety in social interactions tend to greatly disrupt day-to-day life. Those with social phobia understand that the degree of fear is excessive, but feel unable to control it. Although not everyone with social phobia has insomnia, for some people with social phobia, insomnia is a significant problem. This may be particularly true of people who have depression along with social phobia. Certainly, it's reasonable to expect that anticipatory anxiety about an upcoming social or performance situation could have negative effects on sleep.

specific phobias

Phobias are specific fears of an object or situation. Though there are many types of fears, the objects or situations most often fall into one of the following categories:

- Animals and insects (for example, fear of spiders)

- Nature (such as a fear of heights or water)

- Blood or injury (for example, a fear of receiving an injection)

- Situations such as enclosed spaces, or *claustrophobia*

Although phobias are quite common, a diagnosis of specific phobia occurs when the feared object or situation produces an "excessive" amount of fear and when the phobia interferes with functioning or causes significant distress. People suffering from phobias acknowledge that the degree of fear may be irrational or in excess of what's reasonable. Though they may be able to tolerate some exposure to the feared situation, their anxiety in that situation is quite pronounced. Specific phobias rarely interfere with sleep unless the phobia is experienced in the sleep environment; for example, a spider phobia may result in insomnia if the person is concerned that there might be spiders in the room. As with all the other mentioned anxiety disorders, if you believe you might have a specific phobia, seek mental health advice; effective treatments are available.

Chronic Pain

Chronic pain can arise under different circumstances. In some cases there may have been an initial acute problem, such as a sprained back or a serious infection, but pain signals continue firing in the nervous system for weeks, months, or even years after the original problem heals. Chronic pain can also be part of an ongoing medical disease, such as fibromyalgia (the condition that Barbara had), headache, low-back pain, cancer, and arthritis. Chronic pain can also be *neurogenic* (that is, resulting from damage to the nerves or the brain). Some people suffer chronic pain in the absence of any past injury or evidence of tissue damage. Medicine can't always explain the pain, yet the experience is very real. Regardless of the cause, chronic pain can disturb sleep. Sometimes chronic pain and the suffering it causes lead to depression, which makes the sleep problem even worse. If you have a condition characterized by chronic discomfort and the pain causes significant distress or interferes with your functioning, it would help to get a medical evaluation to determine the cause and discuss treatment options.

is your insomnia affecting your depression, anxiety, or chronic pain problem?

Depression, anxiety, and pain can cause insomnia, and insomnia can make each of these problems worse. In other words the relationship works both ways. Let's look at how insomnia impacts each of the three other disorders, starting with depression.

Insomnia and Depression

The following list summarizes some of the major conclusions found in the scientific literature regarding insomnia's impact on depression:

- Insomnia makes depression symptoms worse, and depressed people with insomnia have more severe depression than those without insomnia (Reynolds and Kupfer 1987; Thase 1998).

- People with insomnia have an increased risk of suicide (Agargün, Kara, and Solmaz 1997).

- People with insomnia have an increased risk of alcohol overuse (Ford and Kamerow 1989).

- People with insomnia have a poorer response to depression medications and psychotherapy for depression (Buysse et al. 1999; Thase, Simons, and Reynolds 1996). In other words, they may have a harder time recovering from depression if the insomnia isn't treated too.

- Insomnia can remain a problem even after the depression goes away, which is called *residual insomnia* (Carney et al. 2007).

- Experiencing insomnia increases the chances that depression will return in the future (Perlis et al. 1997).

- In people with bipolar disorder, sleep deprivation can lead to a manic episode (Sachs 2003).

Insomnia and Anxiety

Not a lot of research investigates whether insomnia specifically makes anxiety disorders worse. One possible reason for the lack of research is the assumption that insomnia is merely a symptom of an anxiety disorder. However, we do know that:

- Experiencing insomnia one night increases your anxiety the next day (Roy-Byrne, Uhde, and Post 1986).

- Insomnia doesn't always improve after an anxiety disorder such as PTSD is treated (Zayfert and DeViva 2004).

- Having insomnia increases your chances of developing an anxiety disorder in the future; that is, insomnia is a risk factor for anxiety disorders (Ford and Kamerow 1989).

Insomnia and Pain

This list summarizes some of the conclusions found in the scientific literature on how insomnia impacts pain:

- People with shortened sleep have increased pain (Roehrs et al. 2006).

- Having insomnia and pain increases the risk of suicide (Tang and Crane 2006).

- For people with fibromyalgia, nights with sleep difficulties are followed by days with more pain and fatigue, and a negative mood. In one experiment, volunteers without pain slept in a laboratory and allowed researchers to disrupt certain aspects of their sleep. The next morning, the volunteers reported fibromyalgia-like pain as well as fatigue and negative mood (Moldofsky et al. 1975).

- People who experience poor sleep have increased frequency and severity of headaches and migraines (Rains 2008).

when to treat insomnia that coexists with other disorders

The discussion earlier in this chapter has probably convinced you that if you have insomnia along with other health conditions, you should get treatment early rather than wait to see if your sleep problem resolves with the treatment of the other disorder. You might be surprised to learn that research testing this reasonable assumption only started within the past ten years, probably because the information we have on insomnia coexisting with other disorders is also relatively recent. Emerging scientific evidence tells us that simultaneously treating insomnia and depression results in greater improvement in both depression and insomnia symptoms, compared to treating only the depression (Manber et al. 2008). This is true both for sleep medications and for treatments such as those described in this book. Therefore, we might expect Frank (from earlier in the chapter) to feel better overall if his antidepressant medication were combined with an effective insomnia treatment, such as CBT.

We and others believe that when an insomnia disorder coexists with another condition, such as depression, anxiety, or chronic pain, it's best to take the insomnia seriously and treat it right away rather than wait to see if the insomnia resolves after treating the other condition. By effectively treating the insomnia right away, we can:

- Reduce your personal suffering associated with insomnia

- Improve your accompanying condition (that is, pain, mood, and anxiety symptoms should also improve)

- In the case of the treatment discussed in this book, provide you with tools to effectively address any possible returning symptoms of insomnia

The last point is very important, because as we discuss later, insomnia tends to come and go; that is, it's *episodic*. Following the treatment offered in this book will likely improve your current insomnia episode and, importantly, teach you tools that will help reduce the probability that a few bad nights will turn into chronic insomnia. Moreover, even if for some reason, any insomnia returns, you'll be better equipped to deal with it. Frank was treated with CBT for insomnia, similar to the treatment this book offers. Within a month he was sleeping better. Instead of being in bed awake for hours, he spent less than ten minutes awake throughout the night. This is well within the normal range, because most people spend less than thirty minutes awake throughout the night. After a while, Frank no longer dreaded going to bed, and felt confident that even if insomnia symptoms returned, he could effectively address them.

summing up

- Insomnia is characterized by disturbed sleep that lasts for at least one month. The nighttime disturbance involves difficulty falling or staying asleep, or feeling unrested in the morning. The daytime disturbance can involve distress or concern about sleep, or about the consequences of poor sleep.

- Insomnia is a prevalent condition, particularly when it occurs with another health condition.

- Three conditions that commonly co-occur with insomnia are depression, anxiety, and chronic pain.

- Insomnia can make other health-related issues worse.

CHAPTER 2

learning about your sleep

After reading chapter 1, you probably have a good sense of whether or not you have what sleep experts call insomnia. In this chapter you'll learn more about your insomnia, other relevant sleep disorders, sleepiness, fatigue, and the value of monitoring your sleep in a sleep log.

assessing for insomnia and other sleep disorders

To find out how your insomnia symptoms compare to those of other people with insomnia, answer the following questions by providing a rating that best describes your sleep in the past month.

The Insomnia Severity Index

1. Rate the current severity of your insomnia problem(s):

	None	Mild	Mod.	Severe	Very Severe
Difficulty falling asleep	0	1	2	3	4
Difficulty staying asleep	0	1	2	3	4
Problem waking up too early*	0	1	2	3	4

*"Waking up too early" means that you are waking up before you intend and cannot fall back asleep. "Difficulty staying asleep" means that after you initially fall asleep, you wake up in the middle of the night and have trouble returning to sleep, but eventually you do fall asleep.

2. How satisfied/dissatisfied are you with your current sleep pattern?

Very Satisfied		Moderately Satisfied		Very Dissatisfied
0	1	2	3	4

3. To what extent do you consider your sleep problem to *interfere* with your daily functioning (for example, daytime functioning, ability to function at work/daily chores, concentration, memory, mood, and so on)?

Not at All	A Little	Somewhat	Much	Very Much
0	1	2	3	4

4. How *noticeable* to others do you think your sleep problem is in terms of impairing the quality of your life?

Not at All	A Little	Somewhat	Much	Very Much
0	1	2	3	4

5. How *worried*/distressed are you about your current sleep problem?

Not at All	A Little	Somewhat	Much	Very Much
0	1	2	3	4

Add up the circled numbers to obtain your insomnia severity score. The table below allows you to see how your score compares with other people with insomnia:

(© Charles M. Morin, Ph.D. 1993)

Score	Significance
0–7	People without insomnia tend to score in this range.
8–14	People with relatively mild insomnia symptoms score in this range.
15–21	People with moderately severe insomnia tend to score in this range.
22–28	People with severe insomnia symptoms score in this range.

The majority of people meeting criteria for an insomnia diagnosis score 15 or more.

Write down your score below. When you've finished working through this book and have been using the strategies presented, take this test again and compare your scores.

Before starting the program in the book:

My insomnia score was _____ . Date: _____

After completing the program in the book:

My insomnia score is _____ . Date: _____

We expect that like most people, you'll benefit from the program we offer in this book and your insomnia score will decrease to below 15. However, some people don't improve with this program; that is, their score remains in the moderate or severe range (above 15). There could be several reasons why this might happen, but one is that you may have another sleep disorder, such as discussed next. Regardless of the reason, the best course of action is to seek help from a sleep specialist.

Could You Have Another Sleep Disorder?

Sleep disorders other than insomnia can cause frequent awakenings from sleep and make sleep feel restless or not refreshing. Next we discuss some of the more common sleep disorders that might need to be evaluated and treated, because if you have them, your sleep won't improve completely with the insomnia program offered in this book. We begin with a few examples.

Bill, sixty-three, had experienced several episodes of depression. His most troublesome problem was that he would wake up many times each night. Some of these awakenings were related to the need to use the restroom, while others weren't. Most of these awakenings were brief. He didn't feel rested when he woke up in the morning. During the day he struggled to stay awake, and in the evening he tended to "nod off" unintentionally while watching television. His wife, Betty, complained about his snoring, which surprised Bill because he felt as though he barely slept during the night. Bill went to a sleep specialist, who recommended an overnight sleep study in the sleep laboratory, because Bill's light sleep, frequent awakenings, and nodding off during the day suggested he might have sleep apnea, a disorder in which breathing is abnormal during sleep. Indeed, the overnight study revealed that Bill was briefly woken up an average of thirty-two times each hour by pauses in his breathing. The doctor told Bill that he indeed had sleep apnea, which was then treated with CPAP (continuous positive airway pressure), a treatment that involves wearing a mask or other breathing apparatus connected to a machine that keeps a continuous flow of air going through the air passageways. This treatment usually decreases the pauses in breathing and makes sleep more continuous and refreshing, which is exactly what happened in Bill's case. He now uses a CPAP machine every night, which helps him feel more refreshed in the morning and more energetic during the day. Betty sleeps better too, now that her sleep is no longer disturbed by Bill's snoring.

Anthony was a twenty-one-year-old man with a history of panic attacks who worked as a nurse three times per week. His work shift was from 7:00 p.m. to 7:00 a.m. On workdays, Anthony would sleep for several hours in the afternoon before work, and then again in the morning after his shift, from 8:30 a.m. until 1:00 p.m. On his days off, he slept between 12:00 a.m. and 8:00 a.m. After several months of working the twelve-hour night shift, Anthony couldn't sleep for more than two hours on the mornings after his shift. He could only sleep from 8:30 to 10:30 a.m. Though very tired, he could no longer stay asleep until 1:00 p.m., as he used to do. He also started having trouble sleeping during the afternoon nap he normally took before his shift. After a while he even had difficulty falling asleep at his usual midnight bedtime on his days off. He started to take an over-the-counter sleeping pill, but it didn't help him sleep better. He decided it was time to go to a sleep specialist. The sleep doctor told him that he had a circadian rhythm sleep disorder. The doctor explained that this meant that Anthony's body clock that controls the timing of sleep and wakeful states had become weakened or out of sync with the time he was trying to sleep. Based on this diagnosis, Anthony requested to work only day shifts, and fortunately his employer honored his request. The change in his work schedule led to a dramatic improvement in Anthony's sleep. He now sleeps between 12:00 a.m. and 8:00 a.m., his usual bedtime and rise time before he'd started the night-shift schedule.

A thirty-two-year-old attorney, Mary struggled with chronic fatigue syndrome. She complained of being a restless sleeper and said that her legs never seemed comfortable in bed. Despite shifting her position and moving her legs frequently, nothing seemed to help except getting out of bed and walking around. Her husband complained of being kicked during the night. Mary was sometimes aware of the kicking because she was awoken periodically by her own twitches and leg jerks throughout the night. With her sleep interrupted so frequently, she felt extremely tired during the day. She noticed that the restless sensation in her legs sometimes happened in the evening too, when she was reading and resting on the sofa. Very frustrated about her apparent restless insomnia, Mary participated in an insomnia research study at the local university. As part of her participation in the study, she was the subject of an overnight sleep study in the research laboratory, which revealed that she had periodic limb movement disorder (PLMD), a diagnosis given in the presence of frequent muscle contractions during sleep. These muscle contractions cause brief wakes from sleep that lead to feeling tired during the day. Mary also had restless legs syndrome (RLS), a related sleep disorder that interfered with her ability to fall asleep. It, too, is a disorder of periodic muscle contractions, except that the contractions occur while the person is awake, so it's therefore diagnosable without a sleep study. Because Mary had both disorders, the researcher suggested she make an appointment with a sleep specialist or a neurologist to assess and treat these neurologically based sleep disorders. After Mary began taking prescribed medication for RLS and PLMD, she noticed an immediate improvement in the unpleasant leg sensations. The quality of her sleep improved, and she felt more energetic during the day.

In these case scenarios, the people with sleep problems believed they had insomnia, when, in actuality, they had an undiagnosed sleep disorder that better accounted for their sleep problems. Following are self-tests for common sleep disorders that "look" like insomnia, and sometimes accompany insomnia.

Sleep Apnea Quiz

Answer the following questions by circling "Y" for yes or "N" for no.

1. Y or N   Has anyone complained that you snore?

2. Y or N   Has anyone ever told you that you gasp, snort, or stop breathing during your sleep? Or, have you ever been awakened by your own snorting or gasping noises?

3. Y or N   Are you prone to falling asleep unintentionally while sitting quietly, watching television, or performing other activities? If you're not sure, are there any clues that this might be happening? Clues might include difficulty following a plot on television or having to reread pages of a book (for instance, feeling as though you *missed* something), finding drool (excess saliva) on your face or pillow, or experiencing *lost* amounts of time.

4. Y or N   Are you tired when you wake up, even after a good night's sleep?

5. Y or N   Do you frequently wake up with a headache?

6. Y or N   Do you have to use the restroom more than twice per night?

7. Y or N   Is your sleepiness or sleep problem associated with weight gain?

If you answered yes to any of the previous questions, get evaluated by a specialist for a possible breathing-related sleep disorder. The most common type of breathing-related sleep disorder diagnosis is *obstructive sleep apnea*, which is characterized by frequent, brief pauses in breathing (ten seconds or more). Several factors can cause these pauses or partial obstructions, including your throat muscles' failure to keep the airway open. The brain's failure to regulate breathing can also cause breathing pauses, although this type of sleep apnea, *central sleep apnea*, is much rarer than obstructive sleep apnea. Because sleep-disordered breathing may involve having less oxygen available for your body, the heart has to work extra hard. The heart's extra effort to pump blood throughout your body can lead to problems such as high blood pressure, irregular heartbeats, heart attacks, and strokes. Sleep-disordered breathing can also involve depression. Intense sleepiness during the day is common among people with sleep apnea, so it's not surprising that sleep apnea accounts for more than fifteen hundred traffic-accident deaths per year in the United States (National Safety Council 2001). Though a very serious disorder, fortunately it's treatable. The most common and effective treatment for sleep-disordered breathing is CPAP, the treatment Bill received in the example earlier in the chapter.

Restless Legs Syndrome Quiz

Answer the following questions by circling "Y" for yes or "N" for no.

1. Y or N   Do you have an irresistible urge to move your legs when at rest? If so, is this symptom worse in the evening or while you're in bed?

2. Y or N   Do you experience a creepy-crawly or pulling sensation under your skin in your lower legs? (This is different from a calf-muscle cramp.)

3. Y or N   If you answered yes to either of the above questions, do these sensations improve if you move or rub your legs?

Answering yes to any of these questions suggests possible restless legs syndrome (RLS), the causes of which aren't fully understood. Some evidence suggests that it might be genetic (Winkelman et al. 2002). Pregnancy can cause or exacerbate RLS, but the severity usually diminishes to pre-pregnancy levels after delivery (Goodman, Brodie, and Ayida 1988). Iron deficiency has been found in some people with RLS (Sun et al. 1998). RLS can be very troubling, especially in situations in which moving is difficult, such as on an airplane. Like Mary, people with RLS often also have periodic limb movement disorder (PLMD). If you have RLS along with significant daytime fatigue or sleepiness, tell your doctor.

Periodic Limb Movement Disorder Quiz

Answer the following questions by circling "Y" for yes or "N" for no.

1. Y or N   Has anyone told you that your legs or feet twitch, or jerk repeatedly during the night? If you live alone, do you often wake up and notice that your bedding is tangled, even though you don't recall having had restless sleep?

2. Y or N   Do you awaken feeling unrested, feel very tired during the day, or both?

Did you answer yes to any of the previous questions? If so, consider seeking medical advice. The test to investigate PLMD is an overnight sleep study that provides information on the activities of your leg muscles during sleep. Sleep specialists are particularly interested in leg movements that cause frequent wakes from sleep because they compromise the quality of sleep. A person with PLMD is often unaware of having leg movements or waking up after them, because these arousals last only seconds. Treatment of PLMD usually involves a medication that affects a chemical in the brain called *dopamine*.

The Difference Between Sleepiness and Fatigue

Though the terms "fatigue" and "sleepiness" are often used interchangeably, as we'll soon explain, the two are fundamentally different, and the distinction between them has important implications for your experience with insomnia.

Fatigue: Fatigue is highly common in people who have sleep difficulties; in fact it's often the most troublesome problem for those with insomnia. You might experience fatigue as physical sensations, such as feeling tired or sluggish, or having a sense of heaviness in your limbs, but it can also affect you mentally, making you feel mentally "cloudy" and affecting your memory, decision making, and concentration. Fatigue can negatively affect your mood, leading to grouchiness, irritability, anxiety, or depressed mood. Despite these nuisances, fatigue itself is not life threatening.

Sleepiness: In contrast, sleepiness involves having to struggle to stay awake. Some examples of disorders characterized by clinical sleepiness are sleep-disordered breathing conditions such as sleep apnea or PLMD. As described next, insomnia is rarely associated with sleepiness, but, rather, is most often associated with fatigue. Obviously sleepiness, like fatigue, can lead to low energy and lapses in attention and concentration. However sleepiness is distinct from fatigue in the potential safety issues caused by falling asleep unintentionally. Lapses in attention and concentration when you're sleepy can cause you to nod off while performing a task. Indeed, sleepiness most often occurs in monotonous situations or when we're passive, such as when watching television or a movie. In some monotonous situations, such as driving, sleepiness can be fatal. Many people with insomnia say they're sleepy, when most often they're actually experiencing fatigue rather than sleepiness. We know this because, despite high levels of fatigue, most people with insomnia don't struggle to stay awake and, in fact, are unable to sleep or nap during the day.

Sleep specialists test for clinical levels of sleepiness by giving a person twenty minutes to fall asleep during a nap on five separate occasions over the course of a day. A person who falls asleep within five minutes on most of the naps has a level of sleepiness that causes concern. People with insomnia don't tend to fit a *sleepy* profile on this sleepiness test in that they usually don't fall asleep during most of the twenty-minute nap opportunities. However, people with insomnia *are* very fatigued. Researchers M. H. Bonnet and D. L. Arand (1996) conducted an experiment that showed that people with insomnia were not very *sleepy*. In this experiment, ten people who didn't have insomnia and ten people who did were invited to sleep in a laboratory. Their sleep was monitored using standard sleep-laboratory techniques. For those with insomnia, their sleep was simply monitored. For those without insomnia, their sleep was disrupted to match the sleep of those with insomnia. If the person with insomnia was awake, then the person without insomnia was woken up. The next day, everyone was given five opportunities to take a twenty-minute nap, and their brain activity was monitored to measure how long it took each group to fall asleep during each nap. The people with insomnia were much less likely to fall asleep during these nap opportunities than those without insomnia, whose sleep the researchers artificially disturbed during the night. This study also tells us that artificially induced sleep deprivation is fundamentally different from the experience of sleep deprivation inherent in insomnia. When sleep is artificially deprived, sleepiness occurs, but the deprivation in insomnia most often results in fatigue only.

If you experience insomnia and fatigue, you probably would *like* to sleep, but if given a chance to do so, you would either be unable to fall asleep or take a long time to do so. One of the implications of this characteristic is that people with insomnia are at lower risk of having accidents, such as from falling asleep while driving, than those who are sleepy. To see whether you have clinical levels of fatigue or sleepiness, check the websites for the "Fatigue Severity Scale" (www.healthywomen.org/healthtopics/sleepdisorders/fss) and the "Epworth Sleepiness Scale"(www.stanford.edu/~dement/epworth.html).

keeping a sleep log

Many people who have sleep problems think about and describe their sleep in global terms: They tend to say that their sleep is the same every night. For example, when asked to monitor her sleep every morning, Bette said, "I can tell you how I sleep. I go to bed every night at ten-thirty, lie awake for hours, eventually fall asleep, and then wake up at six every morning." When asked if she napped, she replied no. I (C. E. C) invited her to try an experiment; I asked her to fill out a sleep log for the next two weeks to see if there was anything she might discover about her sleeping patterns. Bette reluctantly agreed.

Two weeks later, we reviewed her sleep log and discovered that on three nights, she'd gone to bed as early as 9:00 p.m., and on weekends, she'd tended to retire as late as midnight. It turned out that Bette went to bed early during the week because she was tired, and she some-times went to bed late when she had social engagements on the weekend. The log also revealed that she'd slept in up to ninety minutes later on weekends than on weekdays. There were two naps over the course of the two weeks as well. The log also revealed that on average, it took her thirty-five minutes to fall asleep, but on three nights she fell asleep in less than thirty minutes, and on two nights, it took hours to fall asleep. Bette also realized that although her general impression was that she never had difficulty staying asleep, on four of the fourteen nights on which she monitored her sleep in a log, she was awake twenty to forty minutes in the middle of the night after initially falling asleep. Bette was surprised, because in some ways, her sleep was better than she'd thought (it didn't take hours to fall asleep every single night). In other ways her sleep was a little worse, because she had occasional problems staying asleep.

Bette's experience with the sleep log is not uncommon; there are substantial night-to-night differences in sleep. It generally takes at least two weeks of recording information about your sleep each morning to get a good sense of your sleep patterns. It's actually extraordinarily rare for someone to have *exactly* the same sleep pattern every single night for weeks in a row. The information gathered in a sleep log often identifies definite targets for sleep treatment. The information contained in Bette's sleep log was good news, because it helped identify what was necessary to improve her sleep.

Can You Really Give Accurate Estimates of Your Sleep?

Terry had insomnia and described herself as someone who worried a lot about many little things. She was asked to monitor her sleep in a sleep log. When she brought her sleep log to her appointment, she complained that her sleep log had made her sleep worse. She explained that it was hard for her to remember precisely all the information she needed to record in the morning, so she kept the sleep log by her nightstand and turned the light on to write down information about her sleep each time she woke up. Terry's worry about the accuracy of the information she recorded in the sleep log made her lose more sleep. Her concerns about "getting it right" and "remembering correctly" are common. However, even if Terry's time estimates weren't accurate, if she continued to record information in her sleep log, she could observe any changes in her sleep over the course of treatment. The errors she might make would likely stay more or less the same over time, and therefore wouldn't be important when she monitored changes in her sleep over time. On average, people are fairly good at reporting their sleep if they do it in the morning.

People tend to do a poor job of estimating their sleep time when they complete a sleep log more than a day later. Your memory of your sleep patterns is particularly poor when you try to recall how you slept in the past two weeks without having filled out a log each morning, which is what happened to Bette in the previous example. The sleep therapist reassured Terry that she need not remember things exactly and that she should complete the logs in the morning, recording her best estimates.

Your mood can distort your memory about sleep. When reflecting on your sleep from the past week, you may focus on the worst night and assume the other nights were as bad as the worst one. When your mood is negative, your brain selectively remembers negative information more easily than neutral or positive information (Matt, Vázquez, and Campbell 1992), which will be particularly important to keep in mind if you currently struggle with depression or anxiety.

The following rules will increase the value of recording information in a sleep log:

- Record information each morning as soon as possible after you awaken.

- Record information for a minimum of two weeks.

- If you forgot to complete the log on a given day, skip it and resume recording the next morning.

Filling Out the Sleep Log

Many different versions of a sleep log are available, but all have several items in common. The sleep log included in this book (later in this chapter), like most other sleep logs, asks you to record information about the following: the number of naps you took yesterday, when you got into bed last night, how long it took to fall asleep, how long you were awake if you awoke after being asleep, what time you woke up for the final time this morning, and what time you got out of bed. Always fill out the sleep log in the morning, ideally as soon as possible after you awaken for the final time.

Following are some guidelines for completing the log. In the morning, choose the column that corresponds to the time you complete the log, and enter the corresponding calendar date. For example, for the night between Sunday and Monday, enter the information in the column marked "Monday," and enter the calendar date for Monday. Using David as an example, we illustrate how to complete the log. The "Sample" column provides an example of how David slept on the night between Sunday and Monday:

1. For item 1, list the timing of any (and all) naps in which you actually slept. If you didn't take a nap, record, "No nap." David napped on Sunday afternoon for forty-five minutes between 2:30 and 3:15 p.m. (David usually doesn't nap on weekdays, so on those days, he'll record "No nap" instead.)

2. For item 2, record any sleep aids, including alcohol if it was consumed for the purpose of helping you sleep. For alcohol, record the number of ounces. The following guide may help: one beer, one glass of wine, and one shot of distilled spirits (so-called "hard liquor") equal one ounce of alcohol each. If you consumed distilled spirits, or hard liquor, enter the number of shots (or ounces) you drank. For example, if you drank two martinis, these tend to have three ounces of alcohol each, so your total would be six ounces. David took five milligrams of Ambien (zolpidem) at bedtime. Although he had a glass of wine with dinner, he didn't record it, because he didn't drink it as a sleep aid.

3. For item 3a, record what time you got into bed. Please note that many people "get into bed" before they intend to fall asleep. For example, some people watch television or read in bed for thirty minutes or more before attempting to fall asleep. David went to bed at 11:00 p.m., watched the news, and then read for ten minutes.

    For item 3b, record what time you began "trying" to fall asleep. This might be what time you turned out the lights, turned off the TV, got into bed, or closed your eyes. Whatever behavior signifies to you that you were "trying" to fall asleep, record what time this first happened. For David this was 11:40 p.m. On some nights David sets the automatic "sleep" mode on his television for thirty minutes and then falls asleep while the news is on. If David *intends* to fall asleep in the middle of this program, he might record a time fifteen minutes from the start of the "sleep" timer on his television. The most important thing here is to make your best guess at when you attempt to fall asleep.

4. For item 4, estimate how many minutes it took you to fall asleep from the time you intended to fall asleep. On Sunday night David fell asleep seventy-five minutes after he turned off the light. He says it's generally more difficult for him to fall asleep on Sunday night than other nights.

5. For item 5, estimate how many times (if at all) you woke up after initially falling asleep. Do *not* count your final wake time. David woke up twice in the middle of the night.

6. For item 6, estimate how long you were awake each time you woke up, and add up all of these times. For example, David was awake for twenty-five minutes when he first woke up, and forty minutes the next time he woke up.

7. For item 7, record the very last time you woke up, even if you lingered in bed longer. David woke up to his alarm clock at 6:30 a.m. but stayed in bed lazing for another fifteen minutes.

8. For item 8, please record what time you actually got out of bed to start your day. David got out of bed at 6:45 a.m.

9. For item 9, if you woke up when you wanted to, or even later, write "0." Otherwise record how many minutes earlier you awoke than you'd planned or wanted to wake up. David didn't wake up earlier than he'd expected. Therefore he recorded "0" as his answer to item 9.

10. For item 10 rate whether you experienced your sleep as low or high quality, in other words, how well you felt you slept—not to be confused with whether you slept long enough.

Now that you know how to fill out a sleep log, you can begin monitoring your sleep tomorrow morning. As you'll see in subsequent chapters, we usually recommend that you have a few weeks of sleep logged before you start implementing the strategies.

summing up

-   Other sleep disorders can resemble insomnia. If you think you may have another sleep disorder, talk to your doctor.

-   There's a difference between sleepiness and fatigue. Most often people with insomnia are fatigued, not sleepy. Sleepiness can be dangerous and should be evaluated by a doctor.

-   Track your sleep in a sleep log every morning for at least two weeks to get a true sense of your sleep patterns. Filling out a sleep log as soon as you awaken in the morning increases the likelihood that your recording will be accurate and useful.

SLEEP LOG   Date Range: _____

Please complete this form each morning when you wake up.

Day of the Week	Example: Mon	Mon	Tue	Wed	Thur	Fri	Sat	Sun
1. Yesterday I napped from ___ to ___ (time range of all naps). If you didn't nap, write "No nap."	2:30–3:15 p.m.							
2. Last night I took ___ mg. of ___ or ___ ounces of alcohol as a sleep aid.	5 mg. Ambien							
3a. Last night I got into bed at ___ (a.m. or p.m.).	11:00 p.m.							
3b. Last night I turned off the lights and tried to fall asleep at ___ (a.m. or p.m.).	11:40 p.m.							
4. After I turned off the lights, it took me about ___ minutes to fall sleep.	75 min.							
5. I woke from sleep ___ times. (Do not count when you finally woke up here.)	2 times							
6. My arousals lasted ___ minutes. (List each arousal separately.)	25 min. 40 min.							
7. Today I woke up at ___ (a.m. or p.m.). (Note: this is when you finally woke up.)	6:30 a.m.							
8. Today I got out of bed for the day at ___ (a.m. or p.m.).	6:45 a.m.							
9. Today I woke up ___ minutes earlier that I wanted to.	0							
10. I would rate the quality of last night's sleep as 1 = very poor, 2 = poor, 3 = fair, 4 = good, or 5 = excellent.	3							

CHAPTER 3

understanding insomnia and your sleep system

In chapter 2 you learned how your insomnia symptoms compare to those of other people with insomnia and how other sleep disorders can resemble insomnia. You were also given a sleep log so you can begin collecting information about your sleep patterns. In this chapter, we'll provide some basic background information on what causes insomnia and how your body regulates sleep, which will be particularly helpful in understanding the rationale behind some of the recommendations we suggest later in the book.

what causes insomnia?

While we don't fully understand what causes insomnia, we do know that it's affected by both the body (physiology) and the mind (psychology). People with insomnia differ from good sleepers in both of these areas. For example, recently developed technology allows us to observe the brain activity of people as they sleep. By comparing the brains of good and poor sleepers during their sleep, researchers at the University of Pittsburgh have shown that people with insomnia continue to have high activity in areas of the brain that normally are "quieter" during sleep (Nofzinger et al. 2006). In the same vein, sophisticated research studies have allowed researchers to tap into psychological differences between good and poor sleepers. For example, researchers in Glasgow, Scotland, found that people with insomnia more readily pay attention to images related to sleep than images that aren't related to sleep (Espie et al. 2006). They also respond more quickly to pictures related to sleep than those without insomnia, suggesting that they're more focused on items related to sleep than people without insomnia. In both examples, it's not clear whether the observed differences initially caused or are caused by insomnia. However, in both cases, hyperactivity in the brain or hyperattention to sleep-related material would seem to worsen and perpetuate the insomnia.

One thing that's clear is that there's a delicate balance between things that make sleep more likely (*sleep-promoting* factors) and things that make wakefulness more likely (*alertness-promoting* factors). Insomnia occurs when alertness-promoting factors predominate over sleep-promoting factors. What follows is a brief review of some physiological and psychological sleep-promoting and alertness-promoting factors that have been studied in insomnia.

Physiological Factors in Insomnia: As stated earlier, the exact physiologic causes of insomnia are currently unknown. A variety of chemicals in the brain, such as adenosine, melatonin, orexin, cortisol, and serotonin, are thought to be involved in the regulation of sleep (España and Scammell 2004). The media and advertisements for insomnia medications often use the non-specific term "chemical imbalance" to explain the physiological aspect of insomnia. In essence, the argument is that either there's too much of an alertness-promoting chemical or too little of a sleep-promoting chemical during the intended sleep period. Such vague terminology leads some to the conclusion that their insomnia won't resolve unless the imbalance is chemically corrected with a medication, but this is an oversimplification. A given sleep medication may work for some people but not others. In reality, both physiological and psychological processes affect the chemicals involved in sleep regulation.

Insomnia also appears to run in some families, suggesting genetic transmission, although the specific genes involved in this transmission haven't been identified (Watson et al. 2006). Another explanation for the fact that insomnia runs in families is that insomnia may be learned; that is, perhaps the family environment promotes insomnia. For example, you might learn from your parents to be overly concerned about sleep loss, and this exaggerated concern about occasional sleep problems makes your sleep even worse. We return to this line of thought in chapter 7.

Lastly, people with insomnia have higher metabolic levels (more chemical activity) during the day as well as during the night (Bonnet and Arand 1995), and their brain waves during sleep have higher frequency activity than those of good sleepers (Nofzinger et al. 2006). Both higher metabolic rates and faster-frequency brain waves suggest that people with insomnia are more highly physically activated (they have more alertness-promoting factors) than good sleepers. Remember that we don't know whether these differences cause insomnia, because it could also be true that having insomnia *causes* these physiological differences.

Psychological Factors in Insomnia: Thoughts, behaviors, and reactions to stress and daily hassles can cause and maintain insomnia. How you think about sleep and what you do to cope with sleep loss appear to play important roles in the insomnia experience. In subsequent chapters we discuss many examples that demonstrate how thoughts and behaviors interfere with sleep. But briefly, relative to good sleepers, people with insomnia have more anxious thoughts and negative emotions just before sleep and on awakening from sleep (Harvey and Farrell 2003). Anxious thoughts and negative emotions promote alertness rather than sleep, and thus can be a factor in insomnia.

Are the Causes of Insomnia Different When It Occurs with Another Condition?

Whether insomnia occurs on its own (primary insomnia) or with another condition, such as depression, the same physiological and psychological factors we discussed previously can cause insomnia. In addition, the other disorder might also cause or otherwise contribute to insomnia. In some cases, insomnia may develop as a symptom of, or a reaction to, the other disorder. For example, a person may begin experiencing depressive symptoms, such as depressed mood, anger, fatigue, concentration difficulties, and feeling self-critical. In reaction to these troublesome symptoms, this person withdraws from work, friends, and family, and spends increasing amounts of time in bed. Decreasing regular activities and spending more time in bed have a negative effect on sleep and often lead to disturbed sleep. In other words, these seemingly sensible strategies for coping with the depressive symptoms have an unintended negative effect on sleep. If these habits continue, we can expect chronic insomnia to develop, and when insomnia develops, it can worsen the depressive symptoms. This reciprocal relationship, depicted in figure 3.1, creates a vicious cycle that can lead to worsening of both the insomnia and the depression. The same thing can occur when someone has insomnia along with an anxiety disorder or a pain condition.

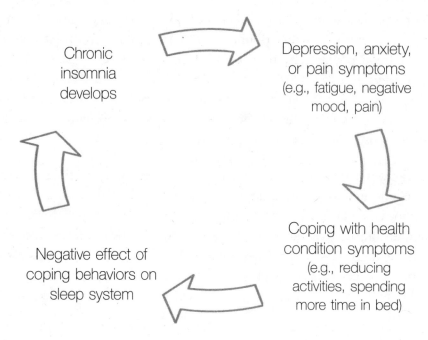

Figure 3.1 How insomnia and other disorders may influence each other

how does sleep *work*?

At the heart of sleep regulation is balancing sleep-promoting and alertness-promoting factors. Your sleep is controlled by two systems that interact to promote sleep and alertness at appropriate times and in appropriate quantities: the *body clock* and the *sleep driver*. The body clock that regulates sleep is one of many internal clocks that control the timing of your bodily systems. The sleep driver system is a *homeostatic* system, meaning it balances how much time you spend awake and active with how much time you spend asleep or resting. Next we'll talk more in depth about these systems to help you understand the rationale behind some of the treatment recommendations in later chapters.

Body Clock: Are You an Owl or a Lark?

People differ with respect to when they feel at their best and most alert, and when they feel sleepy and their bodies naturally produce optimal sleep. This difference among people is normal. For example, you may struggle to stay up until 10:00 p.m. whereas your friends have difficulty going to bed before midnight. As long as your type of body clock doesn't cause significant problems in your day-to-day life (in other words, it doesn't cause you concern or make it difficult to function at work, school, or home), then there's no reason for concern. Most people aren't extremely morninglike or eveninglike, and fall somewhere in the middle. If you're curious to find out where you fall on this spectrum, visit the Horne-Östberg Morningness-Eveningness Scale website (Horne and Östberg 1976) (http://web.ukonline.co.uk/bjlogie/test.htm).

In addition to differences among people, there are natural aging-related differences for morningness and eveningness. Ever notice that babies and young children are more morninglike than adults? Young children tend to become sleepy long before adults are ready to go to bed, and wake up much earlier than adults. Or, have you ever noticed that teenagers go to bed much later and rise much later than when they were younger? Many adults are exasperated by how early their young child wakes them up in the morning, and equally frustrated by their apparent *lazy* teen who won't get out of bed until noon on the weekends. In actuality, their children are probably not trying to deliberately annoy their parents with their sleep habits. Their behaviors reflect normal age-related variations in the body clock that regulates sleep and wakefulness. Attempts to make teens go to bed early or young children sleep in late are likely to fail if you don't take the biological process underlying the body clock into account. In fact, sleep experts have tried to persuade school boards to adjust class schedules so that teens can start later and young children can start earlier. By appropriately adjusting school start times, we could expect improved grades, fewer absences, and better health (Wahlstrom 2002), because our performance is optimal when we're in sync with our body clocks.

Similarly, just as teens experience a shift toward later bedtimes and rise times, as we age, our body clocks naturally shift us toward earlier bedtimes and rise times. Television and movies frequently parody older adults' tendency to become "early birds." Younger and middle-aged adults complain that going out for dinner with their aging parents requires a 4:30 p.m. trip to the restaurant. Similarly, agreeing to a game of golf with an older uncle may result in an unexpected 5:00 a.m. tee-off time. These older adults are no more "obstinate" than the teen who sleeps in late. Those who have a good understanding of their internal body clocks and act in accordance with them (for example, they go to bed when sleepy, and schedule taxing activities when they feel at their best during the day) are rewarded with good sleep and a sense of well-being throughout the day. A mismatch between a person's body clock and behavior can unintentionally create difficulties during both sleeping and waking hours. In some cases it may not be possible to change your schedule to match your body clock; for example, your work may dictate an undesirable schedule. Unfortunately this conflict may result in a circadian disorder, which differs from insomnia (review chapter 2).

In addition to keeping a schedule that fits your body clock, it's important to help your body clock "reset" each day. Our body clocks aren't exactly twenty-four hours long, so there's a tiny bit of "drift." Imagine if your alarm clock lost a little bit of time each day; eventually there might be hours of discrepancy between the "real" time and the time displayed on the alarm clock. Since we use clocks to schedule our activities, it's optimal that our body clocks match the clock on the wall as closely as possible. There are several ways to "set" the clock (and offset the drifting process), the most potent of which is proper timing of sunlight exposure. The body clock's control center is deep inside the brain but receives input from the nerves in your eyes. The nerves in your eyes send a message to your internal body clock about the presence or absence of sunlight. Generally, exposing yourself to daylight during the first hours of sunlight helps to set your body clock for an earlier rise time and an earlier bedtime. Exposing yourself to daylight during the last hours of sunlight helps to set your body clock for a later bedtime and a later rise time (Johnson 1990). Another potent signal that helps set your sleep-wake-regulating body clock is the regularity of the time at which you get out of bed in the morning (Bootzin and Nicassio 1978). When you get out of bed at a regular time, your body clock has a stronger and more reliable beat. Getting out of bed at irregular times weakens the signal from your body clock, which can lead to disturbed sleep. In addition, waking up at around the same time each day naturally leads to a sleepy feeling at around the same time each night, which makes it easier to determine the appropriate time to go to bed.

In addition to these two powerful clock setters, the regularity and timing of other routines, such as meals, social activity, and exercise, can also set your body clock (Carney et al. 2006). If you perform these activities on most days at around the same time, your body clock will have a more reliable beat. Some people with insomnia aren't very regular when it comes to their meals. For example, they may skip breakfast altogether or eat at unconventional times. It's not easy to change habits related to mealtime, but such changes may be important in the overall management of your insomnia. Having regular social interactions at around the same time each day also helps set your body clock. It appears to matter that these social interactions be active, such as involving talking, rather than passive, such as merely being in proximity to other people (ibid.). In one fascinating study, researchers asked senior citizens at a retirement home to increase their activity and keep regular bedtimes, rise times, mealtimes, and activity times (Benloucif et al. 2004). Amazingly, this group of older adults reported that they felt better (experienced less depressed mood) and slept better. As simple as it sounds, keeping a regular schedule of activities—particularly, a regular rise time—produces better sleep and a better mood, because it sends cues to your body clock to keep it working optimally.

To show how irregular sleep-wake patterns affect your biological clock and your overall sense of well-being, consider jet lag. If you've ever experienced jet lag when traveling, then you've probably had some of the following symptoms:

- Trouble falling asleep, waking up, or both

- Fatigue

- Mental cloudiness

- Concentration problems

- Anxiety

- Irritability

- Stomach discomfort

You may have noticed that these are some of the same symptoms of insomnia. How do we understand this? Jet lag results when there's a mismatch between the wall clock and your body clock. For example, if you live in New York City and fly to Los Angeles in the morning, when the wall clock in L.A. reads 3:00 p.m., your body clock is actually set to 6:00 p.m. because that's the clock time in New York. Thus, you may have hunger pangs for dinner when dinnertime isn't even on the locals' "radar" yet. Likewise, you may feel quite sleepy at 8:00 p.m. L.A. time, because your body clock tells you it's 11:00 p.m. New York time. Luckily, after several days of adopting the schedule of the L.A. locals (for example, going to bed, rising, and eating on L.A. time), your body clock will gradually reset itself according to these new cues, particularly because the signals of when it's nighttime and daytime are transmitted from your eyes to your biological clock (Moore 1994). While you're adjusting, however, you may experience some of the jet-lag symptoms we described.

Some people with insomnia experience jet-lag symptoms even without traveling. How can we explain this? Jet lag actually has nothing to do with travel; as we said, it has to do with a mismatch between the wall clock and your body clock. If you get out of bed in the morning at different times, it's as if you're traveling—you have jet lag but without the change of scenery in actual travel. Some people say, "But I only change my sleep schedule on the weekends," but this just means that they travel across a few time zones every weekend. Can you imagine if someone told you that you had to travel across a few time zones every weekend? You might think that this would be stressful, and you'd be right—it *is* stressful on the body. But this is exactly what happens each weekend if you vary your rise time by an hour or more.

Our body clocks are responsible for many important bodily functions, including when and to what extent hormones are released; the natural rise and fall of our body temperature; when we feel at our mental, physical, and emotional best (and worst); and last, the type of sleep we obtain. Under normal conditions these clocks are synchronized. If your core (as opposed to your skin) body temperature were taken continuously over several days, you would see a very predictable increase and decrease by one or so degrees Celsius. For most people, the lowest temperature occurs sometime between 3:00 and 4:00 a.m. Approximately two hours after the body temperature reaches its minimum, people naturally wake up, though this, too, varies among different people and can range between one and three hours (van Cauter and Turek 1995). The core body temperature would continue to rise from this minimum throughout the morning and early afternoon. The body temperature would peak in the evening, and as it began to fall, most people would be ready to retire for the night. The body clock that regulates your core body temperature is strongly linked to the one that regulates your sleep (ibid.). Ideally, you should sleep when your body temperature is falling, and be awake and out of bed shortly after it starts rising. Does this mean you should take your temperature every minute to determine your best sleep window? No. There are simpler ways to know when is the best time to sleep, and we'll help you with this in chapter 5.

There's a window of optimal sleep for each person. If you go to bed too early within this window, you may have difficulty falling asleep and experience poor-quality sleep in the morning. If you go to bed too late within this window, you may have difficulty staying asleep in the morning hours and experience poor-quality sleep. The body clock has the strongest influence on sleep during the second half of your night's sleep. At this time, your body temperature is falling and will be at its lowest point in a twenty-four-hour period. This period of your lowest body temperature in your twenty-four-hour day is when rapid eye movement (REM) sleep is mainly produced (Aschoff and Wever 1981). Ideally, the majority of REM sleep should occur in the last three to four hours of sleep, and there should be a block of mainly deep sleep in the first three to four hours of sleep. As we described, it becomes difficult for your body to produce good sleep much past this time of temperature minimum.

Sleep Drive

In addition to the body clock, our sleep is controlled by a sleep driver system. Sleep drive is the amount of *pressure* to go to sleep your body produces at any given point during a twenty-four-hour period. It's based on how much time you spend awake and active in a twenty-four-hour period. The less active you are, or the less time you spend awake and out of bed, the more diminished your drive to go to sleep. Your body produces sleepy cues when there's a *true* drive. The stronger your sleep drive, the easier it will be to sleep and the more deep sleep you'll produce. The deep sleep produced after long periods of activity or wakefulness is called *slow-wave sleep*, which mainly occurs in the first half of the night (Borbély 1982).

You may be asking yourself, "I'm already sleep deprived, so why isn't my body producing a stronger sleep drive?" Let's answer this question by considering how the balancing system deals with sleep loss. After being awake for a longer than normal period, you typically sleep longer and more deeply than usual. Although you may not recover all of the sleep that you lose, you recover much of the lost deep sleep. You may or may not be aware that you're sleeping more deeply, but if we were to measure your brain waves, we would see deeper sleep. It's important to remember that the quality of sleep is not the same as the quantity. Six hours of quality, uninterrupted sleep feels much better than nine hours of broken, light sleep. So the focus of this book is on producing consistent, good-quality sleep rather than increasing the sheer quantity of sleep. The body's sleep system has the ability to make up for times when you don't get the amount of sleep you need. When someone has an occasional poor night of sleep, the next night the body adjusts and produces deep sleep to balance things out. However, many people with insomnia make changes in their sleep habits to compensate for their poor sleep. They also develop performance anxiety about sleep. If you're tired from lost sleep, it makes sense to think that you should spend more time in bed to make up for this lost sleep. Unfortunately, these habits undermine the balancing system. Spending increased amounts of time in bed (whether resting, napping, sleeping in, or going to bed earlier) sends the body a message that less sleep is needed. Remember, a strong sleep drive is based on how much time you spend awake and active in a twenty-four-hour period. Following is a list of habits that send the balancing system a message that the body should produce *less* sleep:

- Lingering in bed after the alarm has sounded

- Sleeping-in the next morning

- Going to bed earlier than usual

- Reducing activities because of how you feel (for instance, decreasing your physical activities, calling in sick, or canceling social plans)

- Attempting to nap during the day

Although these adjustments seem logical and sensible when you've lost sleep, they can actually contribute to the sleep problems. In fact, in this book you'll discover that these habits actually backfire and end up prolonging the sleep problem rather than improving sleep. So, from the perspective of the sleep driver, what should you do when you've had a poor night's sleep? Nothing; that is, you should maintain your regular schedule. We'll elaborate on this shocking response in the next section.

Did you know that losing sleep one night has a positive effect on the next night's sleep? Remember, the sleep driver tries to balance between how much time you spend awake and how much time you spend asleep. This means that the sleep driver pushes more strongly for sleep the longer you're awake and active during the day, but also, if you're awake during the night, the driver will push for sleep the next night to compensate. For example, in figure 3.2, you'll see that the drive for sleep builds throughout the day and is at its highest before bedtime. This is because there has been sixteen hours of buildup. If, however, in figure 3.3, a person naps at midday, the sleep drive is diminished by the nap and there are only five hours to rebuild the sleep drive for that night's sleep. Even if this person were able to fall asleep at the desired time, the amount of deep sleep would be less than that produced in figure 3.2, which is why it's so important to remain awake and active throughout a day (to build up enough sleep drive to fall asleep and produce deep sleep). Unfortunately, what often happens in insomnia is that people undermine the power of the sleep driver when they try to make up for lost sleep. Because these attempts to make up for lost sleep result in extra time in bed, the sleep driver produces less sleep and the insomnia continues.

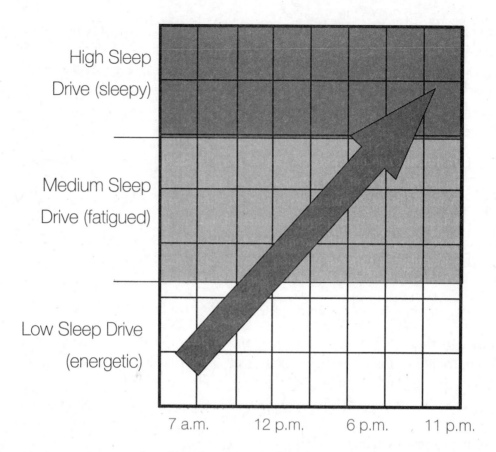

High Sleep
Drive (sleepy)

Medium Sleep
Drive (fatigued)

Low Sleep Drive
(energetic)

7 a.m.   12 p.m.   6 p.m.   11 p.m.

Under normal circumstances, the drive for sleep builds throughout the day until the drive is strong enough at bedtime to produce sleep.

Figure 3.2 Building adequate sleep drive throughout the day

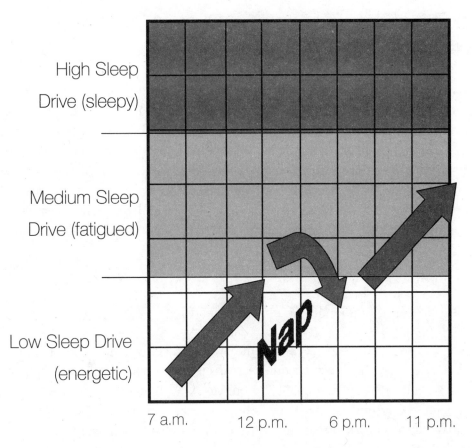

Sleep drive builds as the day goes on; however, napping reduces sleep drive significantly, such that there's not enough time to rebuild enough of a sleep drive before bedtime.

Figure 3.3 Decreased sleep drive at bedtime after napping

How the Sleep Driver and Body Clock Work Together to Regulate Sleep

Generally the body clock operates by sending increasingly stronger alert signals to keep us awake as the sleep driver increases the pressure to go to sleep with each accumulating waking hour. As your usual bedtime approaches, your body clock decreases the alert signals and your sleep driver operates at its maximum level. When this happens, the balance is tipped in favor of sleep. During the night, sleep decreases the pressure from the sleep driver, and the body clock continues to decrease its alert signal. Approximately two hours before you naturally wake up, your body clock begins to increase its alert signal again, and the signal from your sleep driver is at the minimum level. The balance favors wakefulness, and eventually you wake up for the day.

Understanding How Aging Impacts Sleep

As we age, we tend to spend more time awake in bed and less time in the deepest parts of sleep. Because as we age, sleep becomes less deep and we may be more aware of awakenings, we may notice a decrease in the quality of our sleep. Although the reasons for this age-related decline remain poorly understood, many studies reveal that we can help older adults improve their sleep quality using the treatment offered in this book. For example, often older adults believe they need as much sleep as they did when they were physically active younger adults. As a result, they spend as much time in bed as they did when they were younger, even though they sleep less. Unrealistic expectations about sleep can lead to significant distress in older adults, as they worry about why they no longer sleep the same way they did when they were younger. Understanding and accepting that there's some degree of age-related changes can help counteract these changes. We discuss how to do this in chapters 4 and 5.

other "sleep thieves"

In addition to the sleep driver and body clock, environmental factors, such as noise; temperature; the substances we ingest; and inner emotional, mental, or physical tension can all contribute to the overall balance between alertness- and sleep-promoting factors. If loud noises or extremes in temperature disturb your sleep, the obvious remedy is to address them, which may mean using earplugs (or moving to a quieter place, where you can sleep) or finding ways to control the temperature in your sleeping environment. You'll learn more about whether substances may be negatively affecting your sleep in chapter 8.

With respect to inner tension, generally you should try to sleep only when you feel sleepy and calm. Feeling sleepy is a sign that the alertness-promoting system is operating at a low level. The biological systems that promote alertness and sleep are distinct. They don't constitute a single system with an on-off switch, but the two systems interact. As noted in the beginning of the chapter, the alertness-promoting system can trump the sleep-promoting system. This process is adaptive, allowing you to adequately respond to things you view as potentially dangerous that might emerge at night. Therefore, when you perceive a threat in your environment, including emotions such as anxiety, it's difficult to sleep. On the other hand, when your stress level at bedtime is low, you're likely to fall asleep easily. People differ in how they respond to stress; those with insomnia appear to have more stress-sensitive biological systems. For example, compared to good sleepers, people with insomnia have higher metabolic levels and heart rates, and higher levels of stress hormones. The majority of people with insomnia report that they experience difficulty shutting off the mind at bedtime, suggesting that the alertness-promoting system is operating at a high level when they try to sleep. We'll talk more about these factors and give some suggestions for how to deal with "sleep thieves" in subsequent chapters. For now, it's important to remember that good sleep depends on the predominance of sleep-promoting factors over alertness-promoting factors. Understanding how sleep works provides the rationale behind strategies in subsequent chapters aimed at increasing sleep-promoting factors.

summing up

- Your sleep is run by two main physiological systems: a driver system that balances between time asleep and time awake, and a body-clock system that determines the best timing for sleep.

- Match your schedule to your body-clock type. Remember, changes to your body-clock type can occur with age.

- Regular timing of activities that set the body clock (such as going outside, taking meals, exercising, and socializing) will keep your body clock running smoothly (and should help you sleep).

- Sleeping within your best sleep window night after night will improve the quality of your sleep.

- Keeping bedtimes or rise times that vary by an hour or more during the week creates jet-jag symptoms, such as insomnia, fatigue, and mental cloudiness.

- How deeply you sleep is more important than how much sleep you get. Your body has a natural way of adjusting after sleep loss to produce deeper sleep.

- Spending increased amounts of time resting or trying to make up for lost sleep sends a message to your sleep driver to produce less and not-as-deep sleep.

- It's unrealistic to think we'll have the same sleep patterns as when we were children or younger adults, but growing older doesn't mean we'll have insomnia either. Changes in habits and expectations can help older adults produce adequate sleep.

CHAPTER 4

sleep-incompatible
behaviors: tools for change

In chapter 3 you learned that your sleep is regulated by a driver system that balances between the time spent asleep and awake, and a body clock system that determines the best timing for sleep. You also learned that good sleep occurs when sleep-promoting factors predominate over alertness-promoting factors. When considering alertness-promoting (sleep-incompatible) factors, it's important to understand that what you do and how you think, both during the day and at night, have important implications for your sleep. Insomnia is a twenty-four-hour problem, and your experience during the day does impact sleep. In fact some people are more distressed by how they feel *after* a poor night's sleep than during the night while they're having difficulty sleeping. For example, if you feel fatigued and sluggish during the day, your thoughts may turn to worries about poorly performing your job or other commitments. As a result you may cancel your evening plans and go to bed early to make up for last night's poor sleep. As we discuss later, this behavior might prove counterproductive. At night, when struggling to fall asleep, you may feel physically tense, fear that you'll never get to sleep, and worry about how well you'll perform tomorrow. As a result you may become tenser, both physically and emotionally. The tension will naturally lead you to try harder to sleep, which, as we discuss in this chapter, will make sleep even more elusive. This chapter will focus on behaviors and habits that get in the way of good sleep.

sleep-incompatible behaviors

There are many things you can do to try to stay awake: you can splash cold water on your face, turn down the temperature so that you feel cold, talk to someone to stay engaged, or perhaps engage in physical activity. We have a range of (alertness-promoting) behaviors that we can consciously engage in to keep us awake. With insomnia, the behaviors that keep us awake are often hidden from our awareness. Sleep-incompatible behaviors are things that people do that have an unintended negative effect on sleep. Unfortunately people with insomnia almost universally engage in behaviors that inadvertently worsen their insomnia. These behaviors are understandable, though misinformed, reactions to sleep loss. Some might be effective coping behaviors during the initial stages of the sleep problem that, in the long run, exacerbate the insomnia. You may be familiar with some sleep-incompatible behaviors or habits, and others may surprise you. Examples of hidden sleep-incompatible behaviors include trying to sleep in, going to bed earlier than usual, and canceling daytime activities. As you read on, you may identify other hidden sleep-incompatible habits you engage in. We'll talk more about why these and other behaviors interfere with sleep and how to improve your sleep.

What Can We Learn from Dogs?

Before we begin a discussion of specific sleep-incompatible behaviors, we describe one of the most famous, classic scientific experiments in psychology: Ivan Pavlov's dogs. Dr. Pavlov was interested in understanding our instincts as human beings and how the world around us shapes them. He studied dogs to answer these questions. Dr. Pavlov put meat powder in front of a dog and noticed that the dog drooled in anticipation of the meat taste. Something tasty produces a drooling response in all animals, including humans—it's a basic instinct that's not under our conscious control. Dr. Pavlov decided to pair the meat powder with the sound of a bell to see if he could train the dog to drool upon hearing the bell. Over and over the meat powder and the bell were presented together, and each time the response was the same—the dog drooled. Then Dr. Pavlov rang the bell only, and the dog drooled. Why? The answer is that through repeated pairings, the bell and the meat powder became strongly linked with each other. This experiment is famous, because it showed scientists that if you pair two things together over and over (the meat powder and the bell), you need only present one of the pair (the bell) to get the same original response (drooling).

You might wonder how this famous study applies to insomnia. The short answer is that through a similar type of learning, the bed often becomes a cue for being awake. Initially, difficulties sleeping occur naturally in response to certain triggers, such as a stressful life event. Even when the first few nights of sleep problems aren't triggered by life stress, sleep difficulties become a source of stress. Normal reactions to sleep difficulties are to toss and turn, and try harder to sleep. These understandable reactions can then lead to becoming physiologically and emotionally *aroused*. As you can imagine, having upsetting emotions and body tension aren't compatible with sleeping. Humans and other animals can't sleep when in an aroused state, because arousal sends the body a signal that there's potential danger. Animals wouldn't survive long if they weren't able to stay awake when they detected danger, because sleeping when a predator is in the environment could result in being devoured. Emotional arousal signals our body to become alert so that we can take action. It's not surprising then that emotional arousal interferes with sleep. The dangers we perceive in bed aren't related to immediate danger in the physical bedroom environment. Instead, the kind of dangers we perceive in bed include worrying about work, going over our to-do lists, rehashing a negative interaction we had with someone, and, very commonly, being concerned that losing sleep now might compromise us tomorrow and beyond.

The repeated experience of becoming upset in bed, either because of life stress or frustration with being unable to sleep, renders the bed alone, much like the bell in Pavlov's experiments, as a cue for emotional arousal that interferes with sleep. We call this *conditioned arousal*. The bed, bedroom, or whatever habitual sleeping environment you use (for example, the couch in your living room) becomes the switch or bell that turns up the level of emotional arousal and interferes with sleep. This phenomenon may occur seemingly outside of our awareness but is, nonetheless, very important for the reasons we'll discuss next.

some specific sleep-incompatible behaviors

Now that you know there are some potentially surprising behaviors that are incompatible with sleep, we'll identify some of the most important sleep-interfering behaviors.

Staying in Bed When You Can't Sleep

Pete began having problems sleeping a year ago, when he and his wife had some marital issues and were considering separation. He would lie in bed for an hour or two, tossing and turning, and hashing and rehashing arguments they'd had, trying in vain to put these issues out of his mind. Since then, he and his wife have worked out their issues, and their relationship is stronger than ever. Yet, his problem with falling asleep persists. Every night, Pete can barely keep his eyes open while watching the evening news. He feels exhausted and ready to sleep. Every night, he climbs the stairs to the bedroom half asleep, brushes his teeth, and gets into bed. But when he gets into bed, it's as though a switch turns on and he feels wide awake. Pete is frustrated and puzzled. He knows he's sleepy. How could he switch from being half asleep to wide awake every night as soon as his head hits the pillow? The answer is conditioned arousal. During the marital crisis, for Pete the bed was repeatedly paired with feeling upset and being unable to sleep. So, even though Pete didn't intend for this to occur, the bed has become like Dr. Pavlov's bell: a signal for alertness. Therefore, even though he's in a relatively stress-free period and his marriage is stable, he continues to toss and turn for a long time before falling asleep, because now his bed has become a cue for being alert. Pete's situation is an example of conditioned arousal that's exacerbated by a common sleep-incompatible behavior; that is, staying in bed when you're unable to sleep. Staying awake in bed for long periods frequently leads to conditioned arousal, in other words, the bed has become paired with an arousing, rather than sleep-prompting, experience. To unpair the bed from arousal, Pete shouldn't remain in bed when he's in a state of mind that's not conducive to sleeping.

If you want to break conditioned arousal and make the bed a strong cue for sleeping rather than being awake, you have to consistently leave the bed every time you find yourself wide awake in bed. A good rule of thumb is to leave the bedroom within fifteen to twenty minutes of waking up, or as soon as it's fairly obvious to you that you won't be able to readily fall asleep. Similarly, when you're upset about anything in bed, leave the room. Leaving the room will weaken the association between not sleeping and your bed. Once you're out of bed, do something pleasant and calming. Return to bed only when you feel sleepy enough to increase the probability that you'll fall asleep. However, if you, again, feel wide awake, leave the room again. This may seem counterintuitive; you'll be tempted to stay in bed, because you may believe that getting out of bed will make you even wider awake, rendering sleep even less likely. However, although this process may result in some initial sleep deprivation, it will eventually help you resolve the insomnia. A very effective long-term strategy, it takes advantage of the fact that sleep deprivation strengthens your sleep driver system, which increases the likelihood that you'll sleep better the next night. Most importantly, it will help reestablish the link between sleeping and your bed. In contrast, staying in bed will further strengthen the association between your bed and *not* sleeping. With consistent use, this seemingly paradoxical strategy usually works within a week or two. We emphasize consistency, because inconsistency might strengthen undesired associations (Bootzin 1972).

It's important to avoid watching the clock to determine when to leave the bed, because clock watching can be arousing and is thus incompatible with sleep. Therefore, don't use the clock to make this judgment; instead make this decision based on how you feel. When you recognize that you're in a state of mind that's not conducive to sleeping, particularly when it's painfully obvious that you won't be able to fall asleep quickly, leave the bed. You might experience an internal tug-of-war. Part of you will logically believe that leaving the bed will eventually improve your sleep, yet another part will be pulled to stay in bed because it's cozy or because you're afraid of disturbing your bed partner's seep. Remembering the rationale for leaving the bed will help, and discussing it with your bed partner might also help. You might discover that your bed partner doesn't mind being awakened because falling back to sleep is easy for him or her.

You might realize that your bed partner is more concerned about your suffering than about being briefly awakened when you leave or return to the bed. In our years of experience in helping people restore their sleep, we've encountered many potential obstacles to following through with the recommendation to leave the bed when sleep seems unlikely. Understanding these obstacles can help overcome them. Next, let's consider some possible barriers and solutions to following through on this very important recommendation.

Chad had suffered from depression over the past three years. Upon hearing the recommendation to leave the bedroom when unable to sleep, he said that he couldn't think of anything to do outside the bedroom, because he had little interest in doing much of anything. Nonetheless, Chad noticed a fairly clear relation between his insomnia and depression, and agreed that improving his sleep would likely improve his depression symptoms too. With this in mind, Chad wanted to find a way to follow through with leaving the bed and engaging in a relaxing activity when he couldn't sleep. One strategy Chad found helpful was to generate a list of activities that would be more pleasurable than tossing and turning in bed. He then crossed out any activities on the list that might make him more alert. For example, while he enjoyed participating in Internet chat rooms, some of the discussions were lively and would likely increase his wakefulness. Chad decided that lying in bed feeling frustrated felt worse than watching television in the next room. Despite his depressive symptoms, Chad still enjoyed watching television shows that dated back to the time before he was depressed. These TV reruns were on late at night, so he decided to watch them if he woke up in the middle of the night. Initially Chad was also bothered by the idea of leaving his comfortable bed at night. To address this problem, he brought the duvet from his bed into the living room and created a very comfortable space for watching his old television shows. Chad was amazed at how quickly his frustration with being unable to sleep dissipated when he left the bedroom and how quickly he became sleepy again, at which point he returned to his bed.

CHAD'S LIST OF ACTIVITIES MORE PLEASURABLE THAN TOSSING AND TURNING IN BED

Activity	Is It Arousing?
"Chatting" on the computer	Sometimes
Playing solitaire on the computer	Sometimes
Watching television reruns	Probably not
Reading	Not
Sketching on an art pad	Not
Checking e-mail	Sometimes

While it may be difficult to find an activity that's enjoyable in the middle of the night, it's often easy to find an activity that's more enjoyable than tossing and turning. Try devising a list of activities you can do in the middle of the night that are more pleasant than lying awake in bed. See Chad's example in the table. Make sure to assess whether the list contains activities that would make it difficult to return to sleep later (that is, don't do anything that would make you considerably more alert).

Nancy had a different reason for not wanting to leave the bedroom when she was awake for an extended period. She worried that she would *never* be able to return to sleep if she were to leave the bedroom. While awake at night, she also worried whether she would be able to function the next day. Nancy had a tendency to worry even during the day, and was previously diagnosed with generalized anxiety disorder. Though she realized that remaining in bed worrying hadn't worked, she couldn't think of an alternative. Despite reading the recommendation to get out of bed when she couldn't sleep, she wasn't convinced. She tried it a few times but never followed through consistently. Learning that getting out of bed was intended to address the part of her insomnia caused by conditioning and realizing that she would worry either way, she decided she might as well try something different. She resolved to put the strategy to the test for two weeks to see if it would help. To help her hold onto her resolve when awake and upset in the middle of the night, she wrote a note to herself to remind her of reasons that led to her conviction so she could review them if she got cold feet. Our form of this "note to self" is in worksheet 4.2, "Coping Self-Statements," toward the end of this chapter. If you, like many others, are concerned that you might forget your resolve to follow this and other recommendations, it can be helpful to take a moment when you're calm to write down the things that you'd like to remember when you feel upset at night. For example, on her worksheet, Nancy reminded herself that staying in bed hadn't worked in the past. Chad may have written something like, "I'm going to do something enjoyable tonight, so it's fine if I wake up." Although Nancy was nervous about enacting this strategy, she returned two weeks later and said that by the third night, she'd felt so sleepy that she slept throughout the night. Even on nights when she had to leave the bedroom, she needed to remain outside the bedroom for briefer and briefer periods, and there were some nights when she didn't have to leave the bedroom at all.

Victoria experienced insomnia after developing severe pain from a serious back surgery eleven months ago. Even after she recovered from the surgery, she opted not to leave the bedroom when she woke up in the middle of the night, because she thought she should rest. When she learned about conditioned arousal, she realized that the long periods she'd spent in bed had led to conditioned arousal that interfered with her sleep. She spoke with her doctor, who told her that she no longer needed to focus so much on resting and that, in fact, it would be best if she became more active. Moreover, she realized that she could rest outside her bed. Even when you suffer from chronic pain, quality sleep is far more important to your sense of well-being than quantity. Spending time in bed to "rest" doesn't have the same payoff as some initial temporary curtailment of sleep, which builds up the sleep drive necessary to improve your sleep quality. Getting out of bed when you can't sleep also reassociates your bed with sleeping rather than being awake. When pain or other medical conditions necessitate resting, to avoid conditioned arousal it's best to rest in a separate bed from the one you sleep in. Victoria set up a place outside the bed where she could comfortably rest when she encountered difficulty sleeping at night.

Doing Wakeful Activities in Bed

Wakeful activities are things that you do in bed while you're awake, either during the day or at night, other than sex. Before we explain why these activities are sleep incompatible, you might want to complete the exercise on the following page by circling the number that best describes how often you do an activity. Then total all your circled numbers to learn the extent to which you perform wakeful activities in bed.

Was your score 0, or did you find that there are some wakeful activities you do in bed with some regularity? Some people with insomnia argue against the relevancy of this exercise: "Yes, but I've always watched television in bed, and it never mattered before." However, you can probably think of many examples of things you could do in the past with no apparent ill effect that may now have a deleterious influence. For example, you may have enjoyed deep-fried onion rings in the past, and they never upset your stomach. However, if you've had a gallbladder attack, those previously benign onion rings would now upset your stomach. To avoid exacerbating your digestive problems or having future gallbladder flare-ups, you would have to eliminate onion rings from your diet. We would have no way of knowing definitively whether the onion rings and other fatty foods led to your susceptibility to a gallbladder attack (just as we wouldn't be able to determine whether years of wakeful activities in bed increased your chances of developing insomnia). What we would know is that avoiding fatty foods after a gallbladder flare-up is essential. In a similar vein, now that you have insomnia, you may need to avoid activities that you used to do in bed when you had no sleeping problems. Therefore you should avoid wakeful activities in your sleeping environment.

why should it matter whether you do wakeful activities in bed?

The answer may not be intuitive. Wakeful activities are obviously associated with wakefulness; in other words, they promote alertness. Even if you're not aware of it, a certain level of mental and physical alertness is involved in watching television, using the computer, planning your day, and so on. Therefore doing such an activity in bed may further strengthen the bed as a cue for alertness rather than sleep, even if you do these activities during the day. Performing wakeful activities close to bedtime, particularly ones associated with stress or negative emotions, will likely promote alertness in bed, whether at bedtime or in the middle of the night.

Your Wakeful Activities

How often do you do the following wakeful activities in bed?

1. Listen to music:

Never									Every night	
0	1	2	3	4	5	6	7	8	9	10

2. Talk or text on the phone:

Never									Every night	
0	1	2	3	4	5	6	7	8	9	10

3. Smoke cigarettes:

Never									Every night	
0	1	2	3	4	5	6	7	8	9	10

4. Eat:

Never									Every night	
0	1	2	3	4	5	6	7	8	9	10

5. Worry:

Never									Every night	
0	1	2	3	4	5	6	7	8	9	10

6. Watch television:

Never									Every night	
0	1	2	3	4	5	6	7	8	9	10

7. Plan your day:

Never									Every night	
0	1	2	3	4	5	6	7	8	9	10

8. Use the computer:

Never									Every night	
0	1	2	3	4	5	6	7	8	9	10

9. Do some work:

Never									Every night	
0	1	2	3	4	5	6	7	8	9	10

10. Pay bills:

Never									Every night	
0	1	2	3	4	5	6	7	8	9	10

If you study, do work-related activities, deal with relationship crises, or do other activities that are stressful or require a high level of mental activity in bed, the bed will trigger a state of high alertness. As a result you might have intrusive thoughts and emotional arousal at a time when you'd prefer to sleep. Feeling sleepy while watching TV in the family room but becoming wide awake once you get into bed is strong evidence that your bed has become a cue for arousal. The alertness-promoting value your bed has acquired with repeated performance of wakeful activities in it might trigger wakefulness in the middle of the night as well. In some cases, the sleep drive at bedtime is very strong and overrides the conditioned arousal. However, in the middle of the night, after the sleep drive has been reduced by some sleep, the balance shifts and the alertness-promoting cues associated with the bed trump the sleep driver system, leading to difficulty falling back asleep.

So it's important to clearly distinguish between wakeful activities and the sleeping environment, because it will eliminate sleep-incompatible cues from the bedroom and help reestablish the bedroom as a cue for sleep.

Trying to Sleep

One of the main differences between a good and a poor sleeper is that good sleepers report thinking about "nothing at all" and doing "nothing" to bring on sleep, whereas people with insomnia think upsetting thoughts and put effort into sleeping. For sound sleepers, there's a striking absence of effort or engagement with the environment. In contrast, people with insomnia describe a process of *trying* to sleep, which, as we explain shortly, is a potent sleep-incompatible behavior. What does it mean to *try* to sleep? Following are some examples. Do any of these apply to you?

- Get into bed earlier than your normal bedtime.

- Linger in bed after the alarm goes off.

- Spend much more time in bed than you actually sleep, for example, if you sleep only six hours but are in bed for seven or more hours.

- Go to bed when you're tired during the day.

- Stay in bed after it has become obvious that you won't be able to sleep.

- Take more than the recommended dose of sleeping medication.

- Tell yourself, "Go to sleep!"

Spending too much time in bed trying to make up for lost sleep doesn't have the payoff people expect. It's a reasonable coping strategy for good sleepers who are occasionally deprived of sleep by some external circumstance, such as having to wake up early to catch a plane or attending to a sick child during the night. However, this is not an effective way to cope with the sleep deprivation resulting from persistent sleep difficulties, as with insomnia. Consider the following fishing analogy: if you're having trouble catching a fish, although it might seem reasonable to spend a little more time on the lake to catch one, sometimes it's best to acknowledge that the fish just aren't biting today, and try again later.

Sleep is a state that needs to unfold effortlessly. If you remember the time before you had problems sleeping, ask yourself what you did to sleep well, and you'll discover that it's impossible to answer. Reflecting back, you'll realize that you didn't think about it at the time; sleep was something that simply happened. If you don't remember having previously experienced good sleep, ask people who sleep well to describe what they do to get to sleep, and you'll come to a similar conclusion. Good sleep occurs in the absence of trying to sleep. In fact, you can probably recall times when you fell asleep unintentionally, such as in a waiting room, as a passenger in a car, while in the theater, and so on. Reportedly even people with severe insomnia who go to the emergency room in the middle of the night for help after several sleepless nights have fallen asleep while waiting for the busy doctor in a dimly lit room. Several explanations are possible for this medical lore. One is that the removal of the pressure to sleep allows the person to fall asleep more readily. This applies to the person with insomnia who falls asleep as a passenger in a car or while waiting in the emergency room, who is expected to wait (not sleep). The challenge is finding ways to remove the effort to get to sleep.

Let's outline some specific changes you can make to decrease your efforts to get to sleep. To reduce sleep effort, refrain from the following:

- Never get into bed earlier than your usual bedtime.

- Even if it is your usual bedtime, never get into bed unless you feel sleepy.

- Do not linger in bed after the alarm goes off (once you're awake, get out of bed).

- Do not go to bed when you're tired during the day. You can take "power naps" to promote alertness when driving or doing other activities in which drowsiness is a hazard.

- Do not stay in bed when it's obvious that you won't be able to get to sleep.

- Do not take more than the recommended dose of sleeping medication.

- When you become aware of having thoughts such as, "I've got to get to sleep!" recognize this as effort to get to sleep, and read chapter 7 to learn how to deal with it.

Some recommendations we made in this chapter may seem counterintuitive. An understanding of how your sleep system operates makes them seem more natural. That said, following the guidelines we discussed in this chapter might not be easy. To be successful with our recommendations, it's important to commit yourself to following them consistently. The exercises in this chapter and subsequent chapters will help you make the changes you need to improve your sleep. Some readers may find it helpful to first read chapters 7 and 8 to address any beliefs and concerns that may get in the way of following these recommendations.

---

taking action

1. Now that you've read this chapter, set some goals for the week by using worksheet 4.1, "Your Behavioral Plan for Improving Your Sleep." To maximize your success, set realistic goals. The ideal final set of goals would include all the recommended behavioral suggestions in the "Strategies for Change" section in chapter 6, and it's important to do them consistently. However, you may not be able to implement all of them right away. We've included an example to help with this assignment (see worksheet 4.1, "Example: Gayle's Behavioral Plan for Improving Her Sleep"). Gayle recognized several sleep-interfering habits from this chapter and set specific goals for herself over the next week. She managed to meet several of her goals, but it's most important to be patient with yourself and do what you can.

2. Complete worksheet 4.2, "Coping Self-Statements," which may help you anticipate and address potential barriers to reaching your goals.

3. Keep track of your sleep using a sleep log to chart your progress (review chapter 2).

worksheet 4.1 example: Gayle's Behavioral Plan for Improving Her Sleep

Goals for the Week of 5/4–5/10 Check if you met your goal. √	Monday	Tuesday	Wednesday	Thursday	Friday	Saturday	Sunday
1. *I'll leave my bedroom if I'm awake for 30 minutes or more.*	√	n/a	√	√	n/a	√	√
2. *I'll use my bedroom for sleeping only (no Internet in my bedroom).*	√	√	√	√		√	√
3. *I won't attempt to nap unless it's necessary for my safety.*		√	√	√	√	√	√
4.							
5.							
6.							
7.							

worksheet 4.1: Your Behavioral Plan for Improving Your Sleep

Goals for the Week of _____ Check if you met your goal. √	Monday	Tuesday	Wednesday	Thursday	Friday	Saturday	Sunday
1.							
2.							
3.							
4.							
5.							
6.							
7.							

worksheet 4.2: Coping Self-Statements

Some people find this treatment challenging at first. In the beginning, you may notice an increase in daytime fatigue and may spend more time outside your bedroom at night. This is temporary, but it may help to use a strategy to deal with the distress while sticking to the treatment recommendations. Many find it helpful to write coping statements, which they recite to themselves if they encounter difficulty. Because our minds can be pretty unhelpful when we're distressed, making a list of coping statements when we're calm can help diffuse the stressful situation next time it arises. Now, make a list of statements that would be helpful to hear when you're upset about your sleep problems.

Coping self-statement: "I know I'm upset right now, but I must remember…"

Examples:

1. "I'm planning to do something enjoyable tonight, so it's fine if I wake up."

2. "I'll be rewarded tomorrow with deeper sleep if I can be sure to get out of bed no later than my scheduled rise time."

3. "If I nap, I may or may not feel better, and I will have worse sleep tonight."

4. _____

_____

_____

_____

5. _____

_____

_____

_____

6. _____

_____

_____

_____

7. _____

_____

_____

_____

8. _____

_____

_____

_____

9. _____

_____

_____

_____

10. _____

_____

_____

_____

summing up

There are several important sleep-incompatible behaviors to avoid. To improve your sleep, try to follow these guidelines:

- Go to bed only when you're sleepy.

- Leave your bed if you can't sleep.

- Use your bed and bedroom for sleeping only. (Sex is the only exception.)

- When you catch yourself "trying" to sleep, remind yourself that this is counterproductive.

CHAPTER 5

optimizing your sleep system by changing your habits

In the previous chapter we reviewed important behavior changes that are necessary for improving your sleep. Among some of the sleep-interfering behaviors was the idea that people with insomnia sometimes try too hard to sleep and stay in bed when they can't sleep. In this chapter, we introduce a strategy to improve the quality of your sleep by strengthening your sleep-driver and body-clock systems.

Jessica complained that she allotted enough time for sleep but spent little time actually sleeping. I (C. E. C.) asked her how much time she allotted, and she said she went to bed around 9:00 p.m. and set the alarm for 7:00 a.m. I asked Jessica if she ever remembered a time when she'd slept ten hours a night, and she replied, "No—I wish." I asked her whether she thought any middle-aged adult could regularly sleep for ten hours, and she replied, "No." I asked her why she thought it was realistic to give herself a ten-hour opportunity for sleep, and she explained that it was the only way to ensure that she slept at least seven hours. I asked her what she thought might happen if she only gave herself a seven-hour opportunity, and she said she would worry about the possibility of sleeping for only four hours. Jessica's sentiment is very common among people with insomnia. They spend too much time trying to sleep, not realizing that doing so unfortunately reduces the natural drive to sleep and renders the sleep they do get lighter and more fragmented. If you understand your sleep system, you won't have to use inefficient methods such as spending excessive amounts of time in bed to get the sleep you need.

optimizing your sleep driver system

The previous chapter focused your attention on exploring ways you might be putting effort into going to sleep. While exploring this idea, consider the possibility that your current physiological need for sleep might differ from how much sleep you would like. We tend to want to sleep when we're bored, when we're tired of dealing with the day's problems, or when we have something very important the next day for which we want to be optimally alert. We also desire sleep based on how much sleep we believe we need. However, rather than match the amount of time spent in bed to your *desired* amount of sleep, you actually need to match the time spent in bed to your body's current output of sleep. Remember that sleep drive is determined by several factors. The main factor in determining sleep drive is how much time you've spent awake and out of bed during the previous twenty-four hours. Spending more time in bed than the amount of sleep your body can currently produce presents two main problems. The first problem is that as you spend more time in bed hoping to sleep longer, you're also spending more time awake in bed. When you're awake in bed, you exert effort to get to sleep, and feel frustrated and upset. Repeated experiences of being upset in bed can trigger the *switch* phenomenon and the conditioned arousal we described in the previous chapter. The second problem is that spending more time awake in bed produces broken, intermittent sleep, which doesn't allow the sleep driver to increase the drive to sleep. Just as nibbling on food doesn't satisfy our appetites yet diminishes a healthy appetite for food, dozing off or lingering in bed doesn't produce refreshing sleep and reduces the strength of the sleep drive.

Making Sure You Don't Spend Too Much Time in Bed

The following guidelines will ensure that you're not spending too much time in bed, putting too much effort into sleeping, or compromising your sleep drive:

- Go to bed no earlier than you're used to. If you go to bed too early, even if you're very sleepy and do fall asleep, you might sleep for one to two hours and then be awake for the rest of the night. Essentially this practice is akin to taking an evening nap and will therefore interfere with your body's normal regulation of sleep, reducing your sleep drive and weakening your body clock.

- Go to bed only when you're sleepy (and not before your regular bedtime). Doing so will increase the likelihood that you're going to bed at the correct time relative to your body clock. It also means that when you go to bed, the balance of sleep- and alertness-promoting factors is in favor of sleep and will therefore maximize the probability of falling asleep more easily.

- Set a fixed rise time—that is, a fixed get-out-of-bed time—and stick to it regardless of how much sleep you actually get. As we discussed earlier, this is particularly important for anchoring your body clock.

- Refrain from napping, except when you feel sleepy (not just tired) and have to perform activities later that might be dangerous if you aren't optimally alert. In *exceptional* circumstances short naps are refreshing and won't significantly reduce your sleep drive at night. In most cases, naps reduce your drive to sleep and have an overall negative impact on the quality of your sleep.

- Match your time in bed with how much sleep your body currently produces. Following is a description of how to do this.

In addition to the first four important guidelines previously listed, we recommend a process that will improve the quality of your sleep by building your sleep drive. The first step is to shorten how much time you spend in bed and then, once your sleep drive increases and the quality of your sleep improves, slowly increase the amount of time you spend in bed. The important question is, how much time should you stay in bed at the initial step? Ideally the amount of time you stay in bed should closely match the average amount of time you've slept in the previous week or two. The average amount of sleep your body has recently produced reflects your current bodily needs. Though it may not reflect your current desired amount of sleep, it's the amount of sleep your body can produce reliably in its current state. We also add an extra half hour to this number, because it's normal to be awake in bed for about thirty minutes (adding the time it takes to fall asleep, get up to go to the bathroom, and linger in bed before getting out of bed). However, even if your average actual sleep time is less than five hours, your target amount of time spent in bed each night should never be less than five and a half hours. After deciding how long to stay in bed for this initial step, you need to decide when to go to bed and when to get out of bed. Begin by deciding when you'll get out of bed, and work your way backward to determine your bedtime. For example, if you determined that your average number of hours for sleep is presently six hours, schedule six and a half hours in bed. If you determine that you want or need to be up by 6:30 a.m., your bedtime should be midnight. Since ideally you should go to bed only when sleepy, if you don't feel sleepy at midnight, wait until you *are* sleepy. However, regardless of how much sleep you have, always get out of bed no later than your target rise time.

Here's an example: Samantha needs to be out of bed by 5:30 a.m. on weekdays to make it to work on time. Her average amount of time spent sleeping in the past two weeks has been five hours, which means she should be in bed a maximum of five and a half hours. If we count back five and a half hours from 5:30 a.m., this means that Samantha should be in bed no earlier than midnight. If Samantha is not sleepy at midnight, she shouldn't get into bed, because she's unlikely to get to sleep quickly. She should wait until she's sleepy before getting into bed. In such a case, she should *not* adjust her rise time, but should get out of bed at 5:30 a.m. no matter how late she went to bed. This can be challenging for some people, because the sleep drive will increase, presenting a greater temptation to give in and linger in bed, nap, or go to bed before midnight the following night. However, resisting this temptation will create a very strong sleep drive that will likely produce high-quality sleep the next night. The steady rise time has the additional benefit of helping reset Samantha's body clock. On weekends, she must set the alarm and get up at the same time, even though her weekend schedule allows her to stay in bed longer. Eventually (usually over the course of a few days), Samantha will start feeling sleepy at midnight, the amount of time she spends awake in bed will decrease, and she'll experience a remarkable improvement in the quality of her sleep. However, she may also start feeling sleepier, in which case, after a week of high-quality sleep, she can begin extending the amount of time she stays in bed by following a procedure described in the next section. Systematically restricting your time in bed is a very effective method for improving your sleep.

Increased Sleepiness

We should expect Samantha to become sleepier in the first week or two of using the strategy just described. The good news is that her becoming sleepier means that the treatment is working. The payoff will be deeper and less-disrupted sleep. As you start sleeping better, your body may require more sleep. You'll know that you require more sleep only if...

* you're very sleepy at bedtime (meaning that you fall asleep within ten minutes or so),

* you remain asleep for most of the night, *and*

* you don't yet feel optimally alert during the day.

If all three conditions are met, you can increase the time spent in bed by fifteen minutes. If you're now falling asleep quickly and want to go to bed earlier, set your bedtime fifteen minutes earlier (in our example of Samantha, it would mean going to bed at 11:45 p.m. instead of midnight). If the alarm wakes you up and you would prefer to sleep more in the morning, set your rise time for fifteen minutes later (in Samantha's case, it would mean rising at 5:45 a.m. instead of 5:30 a.m.). Stay on this new schedule for at least a week. At the end of the week, determine whether you qualify for an extension, and decide how you want to extend your time in bed following the guidelines just presented. You can continue to do this as long as you still meet the qualifying conditions for an extension. If you notice your sleep becoming worse, it's important to go back to the last bedtime and rise time that worked.

When Beliefs Get in the Way

Though the idea of restricting your time in bed when you have insomnia can seem counterintuitive, it's a highly effective, proven technique (Spielman, Saskin, and Thorpy 1987). If you became anxious when reading about restricting your time in bed, you might take solace in knowing that you're not alone. The suggestion to limit the window of opportunity for sleep tends to provoke anxiety in people with insomnia. Some say, "But I'm already restricted in the amount of sleep I get; that's the problem!"

Let's take a moment to look more closely at thoughts that might get in the way of adopting this strategy. Start by writing down your thoughts about the idea of restricting your sleep opportunity:

Example: "If I limit my sleep opportunity, I'll *never* sleep."

1. _____

2. _____

3. _____

4. _____

5. _____

Now, let's critically examine the belief. We'll use our previous example, the belief that limiting your sleep will worsen your problem. Start by focusing on the evidence against this belief being 100 percent true. Be sure to ask yourself whether you're discounting evidence that contradicts this belief.

1. "I'll never sleep" is not 100 percent accurate; I know I would eventually sleep.

2. Sometimes I spend eight hours in bed and get four hours of sleep, and sometimes I spend six hours in bed and get five and a half hours' sleep. It seems to vary.

3. It's true that the more time I spend awake, the sleepier I feel.

4. I tend to sleep a little deeper after a few bad nights of sleep.

5. Just because I fear I'll never get to sleep doesn't mean that I won't.

6. The sleep-driver explanation in the preceding section seems logical to me.

7.

8.

9.

10.

Given the contrary thoughts and evidence we just considered, write down a coping statement to tell yourself later if you become anxious about the recommendation. For example:

1. Though the idea of limiting my window of opportunity for sleep is anxiety provoking, it doesn't necessarily mean I'll sleep less and it may mean I'll have better-quality sleep, if not tonight, perhaps tomorrow night.

2. Things aren't working for me right now, so I'm willing to be open minded and try this new strategy over the next few weeks.

3. What have I got to lose? I can always go back to my old habits if it doesn't work.

4.

5.

If, after completing the previous exercise, you continue to struggle with anxiety-provoking thoughts about limiting the time you allow yourself for sleep, it may help to focus on the exercises introduced in chapter 7, which offer more tools for changing your beliefs about sleep.

irregular rise time

Keeping an irregular sleep-wake schedule, particularly an irregular rise time, is detrimental to sleeping well. At the extreme are people whose jobs require very irregular schedules, such as rotating shifts. Indeed, insomnia is very common among those whose work involves rotating shifts. Yet even less dramatic variations in the sleep schedule are incompatible with optimal sleep. Having an irregular rise time weakens the circadian clock that regulates sleep. Remember from chapter 3 that jet-lag symptoms mirror insomnia symptoms (for example, fatigue, difficulty falling or staying asleep, stomach irritation, and negative mood). Jet lag occurs when there's a mismatch between the wall clock and the body clock. It has nothing to do with travel and everything to do with a mismatch in timing. Varying your sleep schedule by even an hour from day to day can be the equivalent of traveling across one time zone. Sleeping in a few extra hours can be the equivalent of traveling from the East Coast to the West Coast, and the symptoms can be as severe, creating a jet-lag syndrome without any of the benefits of actual travel.

The most common pattern of irregular rise time is related to the difference between weekends and workdays. When people with insomnia try to catch up on sleep on the weekend, the quality of their extended sleep is rather low. During the morning hours, the alertness-promoting factors predominate, both because at that time the body clock sends waking signals and because the sleep drive has diminished over the course of the night. As a result any sleep that occurs beyond the usual rise time is light and fragmented. Moreover, spending time in bed beyond the usual rise time also negatively affects sleep the following night, because it shortens the window of opportunity for the proper sleep drive to build. For example, if you normally go to bed at 11:00 p.m. and you get out of bed at 10:00 a.m., you build thirteen hours of sleep drive by your habitual 11:00 p.m. bedtime. In contrast, if you rise at 7:00 a.m., you have three extra hours to build an even stronger sleep drive. To summarize, an irregular rise time is incompatible with good sleep because it weakens the body clock and the sleep drive, the two important processes that regulate sleep. The effects of having an irregular rise time are particularly pronounced in people with a more fragile sleep system, such as those with insomnia. So it's particularly important for those with insomnia to keep regular rise times across all seven days of the week.

Ideally bedtime should also be regular. We deemphasize a fixed bedtime because it's more important to go to bed only when sleepy and refrain from trying to control sleep than it is to have a fixed bedtime. In the absence of insomnia and when sleep is in sync with your body clock, sleepiness naturally emerges more or less at the same time every night, and bedtime is regular. As your insomnia improves, we anticipate that you'll gradually move to a more regular bedtime. The regularity with which you complete other activities, such as eating; exercising; starting work, child care, or school; and getting regular sunlight exposure, is also important for an overall strong body clock. People vary in the regularity of these activities. If you tend to dislike routines, focus on a fixed regular rise time, because it's important for optimal sleep. (Bootzin and Nicassio 1978). The timing of sunlight exposure has a direct influence on your sleep, and people's rise time is highly correlated with the timing of their light exposure (Johnson 1990). Generally, exposure to bright light in the evening can shift your biological clock to a later hour, and therefore keep you more alert in the evening and delay when you feel sleepy and ready for bed. In contrast, exposure to bright light early in the morning results in advancing the biological clock that regulates sleepiness and alertness, which results in feeling sleepy and ready for bed earlier at night. If you want to fall asleep at an earlier time, avoid late exposure to sunlight and try to get morning exposure instead. Alternatively, if you want to be able to wake up later (and go to sleep later), you may wish to expose yourself to sunlight in the evening, if possible.

when it's difficult to stay awake until your scheduled bedtime

Some people find it difficult to stay awake until the time prescribed by the procedure described in this chapter for scheduling your time in bed. Isn't it interesting that fighting off sleep may become a problem? The good news is that this means that the sleep drive is high and the treatment is doing exactly what it intends to do. If you're having difficulty staying awake until your scheduled bedtime and you tend to fall asleep quickly and stay asleep, then increase your time in bed by fifteen minutes, as described earlier in the chapter. If, however, you're struggling to stay awake and then you go to bed and are wide awake, or you fall asleep easily but wake up in the middle of the night, then don't adjust (or increase) the amount of time you spend in bed. When you lose the struggle to stay awake until your prescribed bedtime, this extra sleep may diffuse your sleep drive and adversely affect the quality of your sleep. Therefore you'll need to find an effective strategy that will keep you awake until your prescribed bedtime but one that won't then prevent you from falling asleep. For example, if you decide to talk on the phone to keep from falling asleep but then become so awake that you aren't tired at bedtime, curtail or avoid this strategy altogether. The best approach is usually a personalized one, so we encourage you to think in advance about some possible strategies to use. Worksheet 5.4, "Staying Awake Until Your Scheduled Bedtime," may help. Let's look at Alecia's example.

ALECIA'S STRATEGY	Rate low, medium, or high the likelihood this strategy will keep you awake until your scheduled bedtime.	Rate low, medium, or high the likelihood this strategy will interfere with your sleep.
Talking on the phone	medium	medium
Asking my spouse to wake me if I've fallen asleep before my bedtime	high	low
Housework	high	high
Drinking coffee	high	high
Watching a movie	high	low
Not lying down on the couch	high	low

Alecia has several good strategies, but strategies such as doing housework or consuming coffee would make her so alert that she wouldn't be able to fall asleep easily. Thus she should select strategies such as enlisting her husband's help in keeping her awake, or staying out of comfortable furniture that might make her more likely to doze off. In selecting a strategy from your worksheet, keep in mind that the most successful strategies are those that have a high likelihood of keeping you awake until your bedtime (second column) and a low likelihood of interfering with your sleep (third column).

There are other reasons why you might have persistent sleep difficulties despite following the prescribed restricted time in bed. One common cause is worrying that limiting your time in bed will cause you to sleep even less. This concern can produce an alert signal that may override the increase in sleep drive and render the process ineffective. It's therefore of utmost importance that before implementing this strategy, you work through this concern by using relaxation and addressing the anxiety-producing thoughts. Chapter 7 may help you implement strategies that address your worries that you won't get enough sleep. Another common reason why systematic restriction of your time in bed doesn't work is inconsistent use. One night of oversleeping diffuses the sleep drive and renders the process less effective. Sometimes sleep improves if you simply persist with the restricted time in bed for another week or two. Finally, in some extreme cases the sleep problems persist because the time in bed restriction isn't limited enough. When this is the case, you'll need to limit your sleep time even more. Take this drastic measure only if you sleep less than 80 percent of the time you're in bed. Remember to avoid restricting your time in bed to less than five and a half hours.

taking action

Now that you've read this chapter, and have an earliest bedtime and latest "get-out-of-bed" time, add your goal of a particular bedtime and rising time to worksheet 5.1, "Your Behavioral Plan for Improving Your Sleep." Add these goals to your goals from the previous chapters (for an example, see worksheet 5.1, "Example: Gayle's Behavioral Plan for Improving Her Sleep"). As always, it's important to be patient with yourself and do what you can. Ideally, you need to implement this systematic restriction of your time in bed every day. As always, keep track of your sleep on a sleep log to monitor your progress each week. Many ways are available for tracking your progress, one easy way being to calculate the average amount of time you spend awake each week. To do this, refer to worksheet 5.3, "Example: How Much Sleep Is Your Body Producing?" and calculate the value for "2c. Total time awake in bed." Add the values for your responses to 2c across all the nights in your log, and then divide by the number of nights to obtain the average. It usually helps to calculate this value every week or two, because you'll likely be pleased to find that this value decreases over time. It's normal to have a poor week or two wherein the values don't decrease, but overall these values should decrease once you work through the common obstacles for consistently implementing this procedure.

Using your sleep logs from the past week or two, complete worksheet 5.3, "How Much Sleep Is Your Body Currently Producing?" In sections i to iii, you'll calculate the amount of sleep your body regularly produces, how much time you're spending in bed, and how much time you should spend in bed (based on the amount of sleep your body is currently getting). Take your target amount of time in bed each night (iii) and decide on the latest time for which to set your alarm. Counting backward from that time, your target number of hours in bed gives you your earliest bedtime. If you anticipate having difficulty staying up until the earliest bedtime (which may particularly apply to those who have no difficulty falling asleep at the start of the night), you can select an earliest bedtime and then count forward to arrive at the latest alarm time. For example, in Samantha's case, the amount of time she should spend in bed is five and a half hours. She has difficulty staying up past 11:00 p.m., so she sets that as her earliest bedtime. This means that her latest time to set the alarm for is 4:30 a.m. She believes this will work better for her than midnight to 5:30 a.m.

worksheet 5.1 example: Gayle's Behavioral Plan for Improving Her Sleep

Goals for the Week of 5/11-5/17
Check if you met your goal. √

Goals	Monday	Tuesday	Wednesday	Thursday	Friday	Saturday	Sunday
1. I'll leave my bedroom if I'm awake for thirty minutes or more.	√	n/a	√	√	n/a	√	√
2. I'll use my bedroom for sleeping only (no Internet in my bedroom).	√	√	√	√	√	√	√
3. I won't attempt to nap unless it's necessary for my safety.		√	√	√	√	√	√
4. I'll get out of bed by 6:30 a.m.	√	√	√	√	√	√	
5. I'll get into bed no earlier than midnight.	√		√	√	√	√	√
6.							
7.							

worksheet 5.1: Your Behavioral Plan for Improving Your Sleep

Goals for the Week of _____ Check if you met your goal. ✓	Monday	Tuesday	Wednesday	Thursday	Friday	Saturday	Sunday
1. I'll get out of bed by _____ a.m.							
2. I'll get into bed no earlier than _____ p.m.							
3.							
4.							
5.							
6.							
7.							

Be sure to add your plan from the previous chapter to the one in this chapter. The best chance for success is combining all of the strategies.

worksheet 5.2 example: Sleep Log Date range: 5/11–5/17

Info from Your Sleep Log	Mon	Tue	Wed	Thur	Fri	Sat	Sun
What time you got into bed	11:30	11:45	10:15	11:00	12:15	12:00	11:00
Number of minutes it took to fall asleep	30	90	120	15	30	45	30
Number of minutes spent awake during the night	45	60	90	15	45	30	15
What time you finally woke up for the day	4:45	6:00	7:00	5:00	6:15	5:45	6:30
What time you got out of bed	8:00	7:30	7:15	7:45	8:00	8:30	8:30

worksheet 5.3 example: How Much Sleep Is Your Body Currently Producing?

Sample calculation sheet (please see worksheet 5.2, "Example: Sleep Log," on previous page)

Calculations	Mon	Tues	Wed	Thur	Fri	Sat	Sun
1. Total time in bed (difference between time you got into bed and time you got out of bed) x 60	8.5 x 60 — 510	7.75 x 60 — 465	9 x 60 — 540	8.75 x 60 — 525	7.75 x 60 — 465	8.5 x 60 — .510	9.5 x 60 — 570
Calculate the average amount of time in bed by adding the numbers above and dividing them by the number of nights: (510 + 465 + 540 + 525 + 465 + 510 + 570) ÷ 7 = 512. Divide by 60 to convert to hours: 512 ÷ 60 = 8.5 hours							
2a. Total time spent awake during the night (time to fall asleep + time awake during the night)	30 + 45 — 75	90 + 60 — 150	120 + 90 — 210	15 + 15 — 30	30 + 45 — 75	45 + 30 — 75	30 + 15 — 45
2b. Time awake in the morning (difference between time got out of bed and time woke up) x 60	3.25 x 60 — 195	1.5 x 60 — 90	.25 x 60 — 15	2.75 x 60 — 165	1.75 x 60 — 105	2.75 x 60 — 165	2 x 60 — 120

	Day 1	Day 2	Day 3	Day 4	Day 5	Day 6	Day 7
2c. Total time awake in bed (2a + 2b)	75 +195 ___ 270	150 +90 ___ 240	210 +15 ___ 225	30 +165 ___ 195	75 +105 ___ 180	75 +165 ___ 240	45 +120 ___ 165
3. Total sleep time (total time in bed [1.] - total time awake in bed [2c.])	510 -270 ___ 240	465 -240 ___ 225	540 -225 ___ 315	525 -195 ___ 330	465 -180 ___ 285	510 -240 ___ 270	570 -165 ___ 405

4. Total average sleep time (total sleep time for all days ÷ number of days

Example: (240 + 225 + 315 + 330 + 285 + 270 + 405) ÷ 7 days = 296 minutes.

Divide by 60 to convert to hours: just under 5 hours (4.93).

i.   My body regularly produces about 5 hours of sleep.

ii. I spend around 8.5 hours in bed each night.

iii. My target should be 5.5 hours in bed each night (take i and add 30 minutes).

77

worksheet 5.3: How Much Sleep Is Your Body Currently Producing?

Use your sleep log values over the past week to make the following calculations.

Calculations	Mon	Tues	Wed	Thur	Fri	Sat	Sun
1. Total time in bed (difference between time you got in bed and time you got out of bed) x 60	x 60 ———	x 60 ———	x 60 ———	x 60 ———	x 60 ———	x 60 ———	x 60 ———
Calculate the average amount of time in bed by adding the numbers above and dividing them by the number of nights: _____ Divide by 60 to convert to hours: _____							
2a. Total time spent awake during the night (time to fall asleep + time awake during the night)	+ ———	+ ———	+ ———	+ ———	+ ———	+ ———	+ ———
2b. Time awake in the morning (difference between time got out of bed and time woke up) x 60	x 60 ———	x 60 ———	x 60 ———	x 60 ———	x 60 ———	x 60 ———	x 60 ———
2c. Total time awake in bed (2a + 2b)	+ ———	+ ———	+ ———	+ ———	+ ———	+ ———	+ ———

3. Total sleep time (total time in bed [1.] - total time awake in bed [2c.])	—	—	—	—	—	—
4. Total average sleep time (total sleep time for all days ÷ number of days)						

Divide by 60 to convert to hours.

i. My body regularly produces about _____ hours of sleep.

ii. I spend around _____ hours in bed each night.

iii. My target should be _____ hours in bed each night (take i and add 30 minutes).

worksheet 5.4: Staying Awake Until Your Scheduled Bedtime

STRATEGY	Rate low, medium, or high the likelihood this strategy will keep you awake until your scheduled bedtime.	Rate low, medium, or high the likelihood this strategy will interfere with your sleep.

summing up

- The amount of sleep you need is based on the sleep driver system, not on the amount of sleep you desire.

- Spending more time in bed than the amount of sleep your body is currently producing increases the amount of time you're awake in bed and leads to poor-quality sleep, paradoxically decreasing your sleep need or drive.

- Limiting your time in bed in a systematic way increases your body's sleep drive and produces better quality sleep.

- Keeping a regular rise time seven days a week will help set your natural body clock and prevent jet lag–like symptoms.

Don't forget to combine these strategies with the important strategies you learned in the previous chapter:

- Go to bed only when you're sleepy.

- Leave your bed and bedroom if you can't sleep.

- Use your bed and bedroom for sleeping only. (Sex is the only exception.)

- When you catch yourself "trying" to sleep, remind yourself that this is counterproductive.

quieting your mind: tools for change

In the past two chapters we focused on making important changes to your sleep-related behaviors that will effectively address insomnia, including refraining from sleep-incompatible behaviors such as keeping an irregular sleep schedule, staying in bed when you can't sleep, doing wakeful activities in bed, and *trying* to sleep (including spending too much time in bed). We now turn to addressing another sleep-interfering factor: the problem of an overactive mind at night.

the importance of thoughts

In the past many insomnia researchers believed that insomnia was solely a problem of physical tension and that complaints of being unable to *shut off* the mind at bedtime didn't merit special attention. To examine this view, researchers Lichstein and Rosenthal (1980) posed a question to people with insomnia, and they received an answer that surprised many insomnia researchers at the time. They asked people with insomnia what they viewed as most important in their sleep disturbance: difficulties with the mind (for instance, having an overactive mind or worrying) or difficulties with the body (for example, feeling restless or worked up). People with insomnia cited difficulties with the mind ten times more often than bodily problems. More recently, with advanced technology, research from Dr. Nofzinger's laboratory at the University of Pittsburgh (2006) confirmed that the brains of people with insomnia are hyperactive in areas where they should be less active when falling asleep. These studies suggest that mental overactivity is a significant problem for many people with insomnia and shouldn't be ignored. In this book, we discuss two main cognitive factors implicated in insomnia: this chapter focuses on the problem of the overactive mind, and the next chapter discusses how particular beliefs about sleep can be harmful.

---

the overactive mind and strategies for change

The famous author, Charlotte Brontë mused that "a ruffled mind makes a restless pillow." She was correct in that one of the best predictors of whether someone will take an extended amount of time to fall asleep is having an overactive mind. When people complain of an overactive mind, they describe two main types of problems. The first type of overactive thinking involves neutral emotions, and the second type of thinking tends to involve negative emotions, such as distress, anxiety, frustration, or depression. (Thrill and excitement can also interfere with sleep but are seldom the focus of concern.) The type of thinking involving neutral emotions is best described as thoughts that preoccupy you during the day, that "follow you" to bed, such as planning your schedule for the next day, reviewing the day's events, being aware of your bedroom environment, or running an endless stream of seemingly random thoughts. None of these types of thoughts is particularly distressing. In contrast, the second type of overactive mind is characterized by thoughts involving distressing emotions, such as worry, frustration, or sadness. The strategies for calming the overactive mind are typically the same for both types of problems; however, when distressing emotions are involved, we sometimes add a few extra techniques. We'll start with techniques you can use in both cases, and at the end of the chapter we'll focus on strategies you can use to manage distressing emotions.

Leaving the Bedroom

In chapter 4 we discussed the importance of avoiding sleep-incompatible behaviors, such as trying too hard to sleep, and recommended leaving the bedroom when you're in a state that's not conducive to sleep rather than trying harder to sleep. Struggling with an overactive mind is a state that doesn't promote sleep and, thus, a case where it's best to leave the bedroom. Since we already covered this strategy, we won't do so again in any detail here. The instruction is simple: if you're aware that your mind is overactive, leave the bedroom. Don't wait fifteen to twenty minutes if it's painfully obvious that your overactive mind will prevent you from falling asleep; in this case, leave the room immediately. The rationale is also simple: pairing active thinking with the bed will produce conditioned arousal so that the bed begins to automatically bring about this response (often without your awareness). In addition to preventing such conditioning from occurring, leaving the bedroom has the added benefit that most people's thoughts and worries dissipate when they leave the bedroom. One possible explanation is that the act of getting out of bed and walking down the hall will result in becoming more lucid and awake. While many people say that they were never asleep to begin with, often they have tiny periods of light sleep that they don't notice. Thus, you may not be as lucid as you think, and may be more prone to semiconscious types of thinking and emotional states. When you're lucid and fully awake, you'll be more apt to challenge unreasonable thoughts or worries, and better able to quell unwanted mental activity than when lying in bed half awake. For these reasons, we suggest leaving the bedroom when you're bothered by unwanted mental activity. Return to your bed only when you feel sleepy again. You may need to leave the bedroom several times before your mind gets the idea that the bed is no place to worry or rehash the events of the day. Worksheet 4.2, "Coping Self-Statements," may help you identify and replace with coping statements the thoughts that get in the way of following through with this sometimes-difficult strategy. Here's an example of one coping self-statement to help you get out of bed when you can't turn off your stream of thoughts: "I can't shut off these thoughts, so I might as well go into the living room until they stop. No sense in being miserable in my bed."

Counting Sheep

Probably everyone has heard of counting sheep. Have you ever tried it? This rarely works for people, possibly because it may be too boring to hold your attention. Yet, the rationale behind counting sheep is actually quite sensible. People can get information "stuck" in their minds, with certain thoughts or images repeating over and over again, which psychologists refer to as the *articulatory loop*. The mind "says" (articulates) something over and over again. Have you ever had a song get stuck in your mind? You hear it in your head over and over again, even if you don't want it to be there. Have you ever noticed that the more you try to get rid of it, the longer it stays? Try this exercise: Focus all of your energy on *not* thinking about chocolate cake. Be sure not to think about the sweet smell or the way it tastes. Also be sure not to imagine steam rising off the chocolate cake as it's pulled from the oven. Most people find it impossible not to think about cake once it's mentioned. Even the thought, "Don't think about chocolate cake" is still about chocolate cake. Similarly, people with insomnia often try to suppress unwanted thoughts at night, but attempting suppression has the opposite effect: the unwanted thoughts persist even longer (Ree et al. 2005). Moreover, the longer problem sleepers engage in trying to get rid of these thoughts, the longer they're awake in bed. Getting out of bed and leaving the room is one of the most effective strategies to manage this problem, much more effective than trying to suppress unwanted thoughts. Another alternative to suppressing unwanted thoughts is to "eject" information from the articulatory loop by replacing it with other thoughts. In other words, if alternative thoughts occupy space in the articulatory loop, these new thoughts eject the previous thoughts. The articulatory loop contains a limited amount of space, so it's difficult to keep both the old and new thoughts in the loop simultaneously. Maybe this is why people started counting sheep. Counting sheep takes up space in the articulatory loop and may distract us from whatever we couldn't get out of our heads at bedtime. The problem is that counting sheep is boring, so the old mental material may eject the sheep in short order.

Let's try an experiment: Say the word "the" over and over again in your head for about one minute. Stop reading and repeat "the, the, the, the, the, the" over and over again for sixty seconds. What thoughts or images did you notice? Most people report something such as, "I noticed how weird the word 'the' began to sound," or perhaps they saw a visual image of a string of the letters: "thethethethethethe." What didn't you notice? Most people are no longer thinking the same thoughts they were thinking prior to the experiment; instead they're focused on the letters or sounds; that is, "the" occupies space in the articulatory loop such that your prior thoughts are kicked out of the loop. In one study, asking people with insomnia to say the word "the" over and over again actually shortened their experience of wakefulness in bed (Levey et al. 1991). You can try it next time you have trouble sleeping; however, most people find it as hard to concentrate on the word "the" as to count sheep. It's too boring. The key would be to prevent unwanted thoughts from making it into the loop by finding something more interesting to occupy the loop. One more interesting alternative to counting sheep is called *cognitive distraction* (Waters et al. 2003). Following is a brief description.

cognitive distraction

Have you ever wondered what happened to the characters and the plot at the end of a movie, television show, or book? This exercise employs your imagination to do just that. Imagine the plot of a good book you're reading or a television show you recently watched. While in bed try to imagine what would happen next. Use your imagination to generate the next step in the plot or what happens to your favorite character. Imagine the scenery, what the characters are wearing, and the dialogue; make it as real as possible. Much more interesting than counting white, fluffy animals as they jump over a fence, this technique will take up space in your articulatory loop and keep unwanted thoughts out of your head. In addition, it's an enjoyable task, and anything you can do to manage a busy mind in bed is an important sleep-promoting endeavor. One caveat to this technique is to avoid selecting an emotionally arousing story line; otherwise it will defeat the purpose and interfere with sleep. For example, applying this exercise to a horror movie or an intense thriller may be too arousing to produce the desired effect.

Providing a Mental Wind-Down Period

Some people with insomnia work (whether at housework, paying bills, schoolwork, or job-related work) right up until the time they get into bed, allowing no time to wind down from these taxing activities. It's not surprising when these activities intrude into the sleep period. It's necessary to have a protected period in which the demands of the day cease. The appropriate amount of time might vary from person to person, but a rule of thumb is to set aside a minimum of one hour to unwind before bedtime. This period acts as a buffer between an active, striving state that's incompatible with sleep, and a passive, nonstriving state that allows sleepiness to emerge and facilitates sleep.

Some difficulties with presleep mental overactivity may be due to a habit of staying so busy during the day that bedtime is the first opportunity for your mind to mentally process or make sense of the day's events. Bedtime is a quiet period with minimal stimulation and therefore a natural time for your mind to try to make sense of the day, particularly if you haven't already done so earlier. One strategy to fix this problem is to acknowledge that your mind needs to process the day's events and provide time for that to happen. This period shouldn't be too close to bedtime or infringe on your wind-down time, and should be *at least* an hour or two before bedtime. Creating closure to your day will reduce the likelihood of "unfinished business" following you to bed.

You may wonder *how* to process the day's activities. People find many activities relaxing, such as watching television or reading, and while these activities might be ideal for winding down, unfortunately they're not the types of activities that would help you process your day. Come up with your own idea of a relaxing activity that also allows you to think about your day. Some suggestions include taking an early-evening walk, taking a bath, meditating, writing in a journal, or talking to your partner or friend about your day. Writing in a journal about potential problems with a focus on working through the issues at hand may be very helpful. Dr. Allison Harvey (Harvey and Farrell 2003) tested a journal-keeping strategy wherein she asked people to spend twenty minutes before bedtime writing about their thoughts or concerns with a focus on exploring their deepest emotions and thoughts. She found that relative to those who didn't keep a journal, those who wrote down their concerns and their feelings about them fell asleep more quickly. Whether or not you decide to keep a journal, it's important to protect against thoughts of work or anything mentally or emotionally taxing during the hour or so before bedtime.

Constructive Worry

It's very important to set aside a period before bedtime to separate from active daytime demands and demark a period of rest and sleep. However, sometimes when worries arise, they need to be specifically addressed. At such times merely taking time away from demands isn't enough. Worry is, at its core, an adaptive attempt at problem solving, but worrying about things that are out of our control increases anxiety and becomes futile. People with insomnia often report excessive, out-of-control, and poorly timed worries. The least appropriate place for worry is the bed, because there's little you can do to solve problems when you're in bed and only half awake. You may think about a solvable problem and try to solve it adaptively, but the process evokes anxiety that keeps you awake. What's the answer? One answer is to engage in problem solving at a time that enables you to solve your problems in a satisfactory way, a strategy that has been shown to reduce mental overactivity at night in people with poor sleep (Carney and Waters 2006).

How to Worry Constructively

During the early evening (at least two hours before bedtime) devote fifteen minutes to this exercise. Divide a piece of paper in half, and on one side write "Concerns" and on the other write "Solutions." You'll find a worksheet and an example at the end of this chapter.

1. Think of problems that have the greatest likelihood of keeping you awake at bedtime, and list them in the "Concerns" column.

2. For each problem, think of the *next* step you could take to contribute to its resolution, and write it in the "Solutions" column. This doesn't have to be, and shouldn't be, the final step needed to solve the problem, because solutions might require multiple steps. Just write down the *next* step. Write down some concrete and fairly immediate steps you can take to solve the problem. If you know how to resolve the problem completely, then write down that solution. If you decide that it's not really a significant problem after all and you'll just deal with it when the time comes, then write *that* down. If you decide that you simply don't know what to do about it and need to ask someone to help you, write *that* down. If you decide that it *is* a problem but there seems to be no practical solution at all and you'll just have to live with it, write *that* down, with a note to yourself that maybe sometime soon, you'll find, or someone will give you, a clue that will lead you to a solution. The person in the example at the end of the chapter generated a variety of possible steps to solve his problem of needing his car fixed. There was nothing he could do that night, but he listed several possibilities to consider the next day. Any one of all the possible next steps could ultimately resolve the problem, which is more reassuring than feeling helpless about a worry.

3. Fold your constructive worrying sheet in half, place it on the nightstand next to your bed, and forget about it until bedtime. Explicitly remind yourself that you're making progress by writing down your plans and that nothing else can be done tonight.

4. At bedtime, if you begin to worry, tell yourself that you've already dealt with your problems in the best possible way and that you did so when you were at your problem-solving best. Remind yourself that you will address the problems again the next evening and that nothing you can do while you're so tired can improve on what you've already done; more effort at the wrong time will only make matters worse.

An additional benefit of constructive worrying may be less anxiety during the daytime.

Anxiety Management Strategies

The strategies discussed so far might not suffice for quieting anxious thoughts or other thoughts involving strong negative emotions. When worries involve negative emotions, particularly anxiety, you may need to manage the anxiety and tension by using additional strategies. To help you relax your body and mind, we present a few techniques that include relaxation (in this chapter) and an approach that helps you identify and alter anxiety-producing thoughts (see chapter 7).

Tina was very frustrated as she related her story about how her insomnia began. She had a degenerative disk condition resulting in chronic back pain that made it seem impossible to get comfortable in bed because it hurt to lie down. Tina diligently followed the insomnia treatment recommendations but continued to struggle with pain, frustration, and an overactive mind whenever she got into bed. Her physiotherapist added a yoga routine to her physical therapy regimen to strengthen her back muscles and better support the degenerative disks. Yoga was initially difficult for Tina but became easier over time. The largest improvement in adding the yoga, she noted, was not related to her back problem. Instead, Tina discovered that overall, she was more calm in body and spirit in the evening and at nighttime. She continued to practice yoga and, with the addition of other tools for managing insomnia, made remarkable improvements in her sleep.

People differ in how they respond to various relaxation strategies. Some say, "I've tried relaxation, but I'm not good at it." These people probably tried a technique that didn't match them well, so they quit trying without considering the possibility that another technique might provide tremendous benefits. We encourage you to try a variety of relaxation methods, approaching each with an open mind so you can truly evaluate each one. This approach will likely help you find a beneficial method. Realize that like any skill, continued practice will improve your performance and increase the benefits you derive from it. People who have the greatest difficulty using a relaxation method are probably more tense, revved, or anxious than most, and may need to persist until they find a method that works.

Still, it's unlikely that relaxation alone will suffice for treating chronic insomnia, because relaxation doesn't address strengthening the body clock and sleep driver. However, some people may need a relaxation strategy to augment the other aspects of treatment described in this book, because their physical or emotional tension, or both need to be addressed directly. Next we briefly describe a relaxation technique you might find helpful. For a more thorough description of relaxation and stress management strategies, refer to other relaxation and stress sources at www.newharbinger.com, or seek help from a mental health provider.

relaxation

Relaxation improves sleep, but if you use it alone, you may experience fewer benefits than those derived from changing your sleep behaviors, as presented in chapters 4 and 5. Next we present a how-to guide for one form of relaxation, *progressive muscle relaxation* (PMR), because it has been used extensively with insomnia patients. Even though it is focused on muscle relaxation, when done correctly it produces general relaxation, including a quieter mind. This doesn't mean that this technique would be the most effective approach for you. No matter which relaxation strategy you use, any reduction in muscle tension, heart rate, respiration, or mental overactivity will likely help with your overall insomnia management program. Some people use breathing-based relaxation methods such as slow diaphragmatic breathing or breath meditation, some focus on visualizing a pleasant and relaxing image, some use meditation, and some use calming yoga poses. There doesn't appear to be one form of relaxation that's superior to another with respect to improving your sleep or general sense of well-being. Pick a strategy that appeals to you personally, and use it. Remember, relaxation is a skill that can be learned and needs to be practiced. It's benefits will extend beyond improvement of sleep.

Ideally learn to self-administer the relaxation procedure that you use, because when we need to relax most, we often have no access to a teacher or relaxation CD. Initially you might want to use an audio guide for your practice, but with practice, you can learn to self-administer the relaxation routine. Many relaxation tapes are available (see www.newharbinger.com), so choose one than appeals to you.

Progressive Muscle Relaxation

PMR has been tested many times in people with insomnia and appears to lead to modest sleep improvements. In addition to relaxing the body, PMR may decrease the intrusion of unwanted thoughts as you try to fall asleep (Borkovec and Hennings 1978). PMR is most effective when approached as a practice; that is, something you do every day. You can purchase a CD or read through the following script and then, using a handheld recorder or your computer to burn a

CD, recording your own script to use during subsequent practice. Remember, once you've mastered the technique, you can use it without the guide of a CD.

Begin by finding a comfortable place to lie down. If pain is an issue for you, be sure to leave some extra time to arrange a comfortable place to lie down for about twenty minutes, appropriately propping your body to minimize discomfort. The idea behind PMR is that you focus on the contrast between tensing and releasing different muscle groups. The tension or flexion should build until your muscle is as tense as you can get it without straining. Hold the tension for about seven to eight seconds, focusing on its sensation, and then fully release the muscle until it's as limp as possible. It's crucial to focus on the extremes in sensing tension and relaxation. Some people find it helpful to say, "Relax," or to exhale as they relax their muscles. Stay as focused as possible on this difference, but if your mind wanders, bring your attention gently back to the exercise without judging yourself. Continued practice without judgment will improve your ability to stay focused on the exercise and deepen your ability to relax during the practice:

1. Lie down in a comfortable position.

2. Focus on your right foot as you slowly breathe in and out. Now flex the muscles of your right foot by curling your right toes downward. You'll notice that your ankle is flexed too. Hold the tension as tightly as possible without producing a cramp. Hold it for seven seconds. Then exhale and quickly release all of the tension. Your toes uncurl, your foot comes toward your body, and your ankle settles to a comfortable, natural pose. Your arch is warm with sensations of the release of tension.

3. Now focus farther up your right leg on your calf. Flex your right calf by curling your toes upward and isolating the calf muscles. If you sense a cramp, release slightly. Hold for seven seconds. Then exhale and release. Focus on the difference between the tension and the release.

4. Now focus on the upper part of your right leg. When flexing this long, strong muscle, you'll likely notice some tightening in your knee, hip, and buttock. Flex and hold for seven seconds. Then feel a sense of release on the exhalation. Contrast it with the feeling of tension you experienced when you tensed the muscles.

5. Now do the same thing all over again with your left leg. Focus your attention on your left foot as you slowly breathe in and out. Now flex the muscles of your left foot by curling your left toes downward and flexing the muscles around your ankle. Hold the tension as tightly as possible without producing a cramp. Hold it for seven seconds. Then exhale and quickly release all of the tension. Your toes uncurl and your ankle settles to a comfortable, natural pose. The arch of your left foot is warm with sensations of release.

6.   Now focus farther up your left leg on your calf. Flex your left calf by curling your toes upward and isolating the calf muscles. If you sense a cramp, release slightly. Hold for seven seconds. Then exhale and release. Focus on the difference between the tension and the release.

7.   Now focus on the upper part of your left leg. To flex this long, strong muscle, you'll likely notice some tightening in your knee, hip, and buttock. Flex and hold for seven seconds. Then feel a sense of release on the exhalation.

8.   Now focus on your abdomen. If you have trouble flexing your stomach muscles, suck them in and hold firmly for seven seconds. Hold, hold, hold, and then release. Feel your stomach muscles relax with the gush of air released on the exhale. Feel your abdominal muscles spread upward and along your sides as they relax.

9.   Sense your right hand. Now clench it into a fist as tightly as comfortably possible, and hold for seven seconds. Then release, allowing your fingers to slowly unfurl and become limp.

10. Now focus on the muscles on the inside of your right forearm, and flex them by flexing your wrist upward. Don't overdo it. Simply flex it as much as comfortably possible for seven seconds and then blow out relaxation with the exhale.

11. Move up your right arm and focus on the bicep. You can flex it by "making a muscle"; that is, bending at the elbow and pulling the forearm up toward the shoulder. Now hold this muscle and feel how round it gets when tensed. Then release. Bring your forearm back down, and feel how the bicep muscle elongates when relaxed.

12. Switch to the other side of your body and focus on your left hand. Clench it into a fist as tightly as comfortably possible, and hold for seven seconds. Then release, allowing your fingers to slowly unfurl and fall.

13. Focus on the muscles on the inside of your left forearm. Flex them by flexing your wrist upward. Hold it outstretched and flexed for seven seconds and then relax. Focus on the tingling warmth of relaxation in your forearm.

14.   Move your attention to your left arm and focus on the bicep. As you did with the right side, flex it by pulling the forearm up toward the shoulder. Hold this muscle for seven seconds and feel how round it gets when tensed. Then release. Bring your forearm back down and feel how the bicep muscle elongates when relaxed.

15. Let's move our focus to one of the tenser areas for most people. Tense your neck and shoulders by raising your shoulders up toward your ears and then rolling your shoulder blades back toward each other. Now flex your neck muscles by pressing your head toward your back. Your chest will arch upward as you do this. Be gentle, but hold the tension for seven seconds. Then focus all your attention on the sense of release. The center of your back will press toward the surface you're lying on, as will the base of your head. Focus on the warmth and tingling as these muscles relax.

16. Scrunch your face muscles by squinting your eyes and pursing your lips as you tighten your cheeks into a close-mouthed smile. Hold this pose for seven seconds. Then release.

17. Last, tighten your forehead by raising your eyebrows as high as possible. Hold the pose for seven seconds. Then release. Feel your eyebrows and forehead muscles smoothing into relaxation.

Practice PMR every day. With continued practice you'll experience a gradual reduction in your usual degree of muscle tension. In addition, throughout the day, when you notice tension in a particular muscle group, tense and hold that muscle group, and then release it. PMR teaches you to relax your muscles. With time, people become so adept at this technique that they can more readily notice tension and fully relax a tense muscle without having to first focus on tensing it. They simply say, "Release" or "Relax," and then exhale the tension away. However, it takes quite a bit of practice to develop this briefer skill.

Barriers to Relaxation Practice: Potential barriers to adopting a PMR practice include certain physical conditions, difficulty making the time, motivational difficulties, boredom while listening to the CD, and anxiety about relaxation. Let's focus on each of these potential barriers and how to overcome them. Certain physical problems make it difficult to isolate specific muscle groups, or painful to tense some muscles. In this case we advise speaking with your doctor before embarking on PMR to ensure that it's a medically approved activity for you. Perhaps your doctor won't want you to do this exercise, or will want you to omit or substitute specific muscle groups to avoid injury. Though it's rare that a doctor advises against PMR, it's best to ask. Difficulty finding twenty minutes for practice each day is a common problem in our modern, busy lives. Boredom with the practice can also reduce the likelihood that we'll do it. Conviction in the importance of this practice is essential to overcome both boredom and time limitations. Increased awareness of the tension you carry will help motivate you to practice. To further help you deal with issues of boredom, motivation, and time, list the costs and benefits of carving out twenty minutes a day to practice. Consider making a list similar to the following one.

Costs of a Relaxation Practice	Benefits of a Relaxation Practice
• It takes too much time. I could get some other work done in twenty minutes.	• I'm tired of feeling tense all the time, and it might bring some relief.
• The CD is so boring.	• Maybe getting this tension under control will help me sleep better.
• I'd rather watch TV; that's relaxing.	• It would be nice to do something just for me, for my own well-being.
	• I feel really good after I do it.
	• I need to do something; I know I need to make a change.

It's also possible that now is simply not the right time for you to make this important change. Some people are at a stage in their lives wherein they recognize that they need to make a change but aren't quite ready to take the next step. It's far better to accept that this is where you are without judging yourself than to engage in disparaging self-talk, such as, "I'm lazy for not doing this." This type of self-talk isn't helpful and will only make the situation worse. Saying something like this to someone you love wouldn't be very motivating, would it?

One final barrier that merits discussion is experiencing anxiety about relaxing or feeling more tension when trying to relax. Sometimes the anxiety about relaxing relates to perfectionism and a focus on the outcome, ignoring the fact that relaxation is a process. To believe that there's a single "right" way to complete relaxation exercises is misleading. It's a fixation on outcome that doesn't allow the process of relaxation to unfold. To overcome anxieties about relaxing, it helps to remember that tension levels wax and wane, and being able to recognize tension is the first step in the relaxation process. The process of relaxation involves reduction of tension rather than absence of all tension. Therefore, the moment you realize that you have more tension than usual is a pivotal moment that allows you to move toward lessening the tension. Accepting where you are at a particular moment allows you the freedom to move to a less tense moment. Thoughts such as, "I can't release that muscle fully," "I don't think I held that for seven seconds," or "I can't seem to isolate that muscle" reflect unnecessary perfectionism that will likely further increase rather than decrease tension. The great thing about relaxation is that it doesn't have to be perfect; it's a *practice*, an ongoing process. Feeling an impulse to fix or control the relaxation practice is a sign that persisting with your relaxation practice would particularly help you. Relaxation practice can help you let go of the impulse to "get it right" and to accept wherever your practice takes you. When you notice a perfectionistic or critical voice creeping into your practice, gently acknowledge that you're having a critical thought and then bring your focus back to the practice. Remind yourself that your practice is okay as it is right now.

Anxiety related to relaxing can sometimes result from the surfacing of previously ignored or suppressed feelings that the quiet, relaxed state allow to come into awareness. Some people react to this experience by avoiding relaxation practice, but the same unwanted feelings are prone to resurface when you get into bed or as you lie awake in the middle of the night. It may help to deal with them during the day to reduce the likelihood that they'll interfere with your sleep at night. Remind yourself that your feelings and the thoughts that accompany them are not dangerous. You can work through them as you practice relaxation. In the beginning, you can try shorter relaxation sessions, but don't try to escape the feelings that emerge. Instead stay with them and tolerate them. With repeated practice, your anxiety about relaxing will lessen, and you'll be able to increase your practice time. Fighting against or trying to suppress feelings often intensifies the feelings and makes them more likely to come up again. Breathing deeply and acknowledging (without judging) the sensation of the feelings that emerge will make it easier to manage them. For example, when you notice signs of anxiety, tell yourself in your kindest voice: "I notice that I have butterflies in my stomach. That's okay. I'll bring my attention back to my breath. My chest is rising and falling..." Focusing on thoughts such as, "I don't want this," may prolong the experience. Your willingness to experience feelings paradoxically makes them easier to bear. You might want to try another relaxation method that might be equally or more effective for you and may not produce unwanted experiences. For that reason we encourage you to experiment with different relaxation methods to find one that works best for you. Other relaxation methods to consider include a warm bath, autogenic relaxation, slow diaphragmatic breathing, imagery, relaxing music, meditation, massage, acupuncture, and yoga. Extreme cases of relaxation-related anxiety may require the assistance of a professional psychotherapist. Even if you don't have relaxation-related anxiety, if you believe that anxiety and tension contribute prominently to your insomnia, it may be best to enlist the help of an anxiety expert. Besides anxiety-focused psychotherapy, effective anxiety treatments can include prescription medications. There's no reason to expect that you couldn't use our insomnia recommendations and an outside anxiety treatment simultaneously.

taking action

1. Add whatever exercises in this chapter you intend to use to address an overactive mind to worksheet 4.1, "Your Behavioral Plan for Improving Your Sleep."

2. Monitor your progress using your sleep log (see chapter 2).

3. If you chose to include a relaxation practice in your treatment plan, use worksheet 6.2, "Relaxation Log" to track your practice and how relaxed you are before and after each practice. Remember you're looking for progress, not perfection.

worksheet 6.1 example: Constructive Worrying

Concerns	Solutions
I need to get the car fixed now, but I won't have money until I get paid in two more weeks.	• I can call my friend tomorrow morning and see if I can borrow some money. • I don't actually know how much it will cost, so I may have enough credit on my credit card. • I'll talk to the garage tomorrow about the cost and possible payment options. Maybe they'll accept a later payment? • I can look at the public transit schedule after I finish this exercise. • I can phone the payroll department and ask if there's a way to receive an advance.

worksheet 6.1: Constructive Worrying

Concerns	Solutions

worksheet 6.2: Relaxation Log

My goal this week is to practice _____ times for _____ minutes each.

Day of the Week	Did You Practice? Y = Yes N = No	Tension Before Practice Rate on a scale from 0 to 5 in which 0 = no tension, and 5 = extremely tense.	Tension After Practice Rate on a scale from 0 to 5 in which 0 = no tension, and 5 = extremely tense.

summing up

This chapter focused on the common problem of an overactive mind. If unwanted thoughts are keeping you awake, try the following strategies:

- Leave the bedroom when unwanted thoughts are bothering you.

- Use cognitive distraction: take charge of your "articulatory loop" by imagining the next developments in characters and the plot of a movie you've seen recently or a book you're reading.

- Create a mental wind-down period: anticipate your mind's need to process the day's events by providing a demands-free period *at least* an hour or two before bedtime.

- If you tend to worry or solve problems while in bed, schedule some structured worry time in the early evening to address concerns when your mind is better able to solve problems adaptively (use worksheet 6.1, "Constructive Worrying," to help guide this process).

- Start a daily relaxation practice for a greater sense of well-being, fewer intrusions of unwanted thoughts into your bedroom, less stress, less muscle tension, and sounder sleep.

CHAPTER 7

when thinking about sleep gets in the way of sleep

In the previous chapter we introduced some ways to manage an overactive mind to help you sleep. In this chapter we'll continue considering the importance of mental processes in getting good sleep. Our focus will be on the ways in which people with insomnia think about sleep and how replacing these thoughts with more helpful thoughts can actually improve sleep.

thoughts, feelings, and behaviors: how changes in one area affect the others

It may seem strange at first to consider that what you do, how you feel, and what you think have such a large impact on how you sleep, but it's true. Setting sleep aside for the moment, imagine that you've inadvertently hit your thumb very hard with a hammer. The pain is so intense that all your attention becomes focused on it. Besides pain, you also experience frustration and anger.

You're completely consumed with the thought, "Please stop hurting!" Nothing else can hold your attention. But then you notice that the person next to you is holding a giant check and telling you that because you were the millionth customer in the hardware store, you've just won a million dollars. A smile emerges on your face and your attention turns toward this enormous check. What will you spend the money on? How does your thumb feel now? Did you forget about it for a moment? Sure, your thumb still hurts, but it's now a dull throb in the background of your mind. Your attention is occupied for the moment by this exciting turn of events. What can we learn from this scenario? Were you never in pain to begin with? Of course, not! The pain was and is real. The fact is that what you think, where your attention is, and what you do greatly influence how you feel.

Now let's return to thinking about insomnia. Suppose you had a fight with your spouse before getting into bed. You feel very angry but are determined to try to get some sleep. What would you predict the next thirty minutes to be like for you? Most people find it very difficult to fall asleep quickly when bothered by emotionally charged thoughts. Now imagine that your partner turns over and sincerely apologizes. Your anger fades. Would you now likely have a different experience in the next thirty minutes?

Insomnia, like pain, involves complex interactions among what you do, how you feel, and what you think. We already discussed some ways in which your behavior affects your chances of falling asleep. For example, going to bed too early and feeling frustrated that you can't immediately get to sleep reduces your chances of falling asleep quickly. We discussed how changing behaviors that interfere with the sleep driver or body clock can effectively produce long-lasting recovery. We also touched upon the thoughts that lead us to increase our sleep effort and the behaviors that interfere with sleep. In this chapter we'll revisit and address sleep-interfering beliefs and thoughts, because they're an important part of the overall management of your insomnia. Research shows that people whose sleep-related beliefs became more realistic and flexible with the type of treatment described in this book spend less time awake in the middle of the night, gain more confidence in their ability to sleep, and rate their insomnia symptoms as less severe than those whose beliefs about sleep remained unaltered (Carney and Edinger 2006).

Thoughts, Behaviors, and Feelings Tend to Be Consistent

Your thoughts and behaviors will likely be consistent with your current emotional state. If you feel anxious, you'll likely have an anxious thought, behave in an anxious way, and avoid the thing you're afraid of. Similarly, if you feel pain, you'll likely think about your pain and engage in pain-related behaviors, for instance, resting the sore area. When you think depressing thoughts, are you as likely to take on new projects as when you think more positively? Probably not. It's difficult to do new things when you're facing depressing and deflating thoughts. This same principle applies to insomnia. Try the following exercise to see the connections between having a distressing thought and how you might subsequently feel, think, or behave.

If you think, "I'll *never* get to sleep tonight," how would you most likely feel?

- ☐ Happy

- ☐ Frustrated

- ☐ Upset

- ☐ Bored

- ☐ Scared

- ☐ Other: _____

What kinds of thoughts or images would most likely follow from the thought, "I'll *never* get to sleep tonight"?

- ☐ "Ugh, why do I keep having these problems?"

- ☐ "I'm sure I'll get to sleep eventually."

- ☐ Mental image of yourself tossing and turning in bed.

- ☐ "Oh no, I have a big day tomorrow."

- ☐ "Well, now I'll never get to sleep for sure."

- ☐ Other: _____

What action would you most likely take after thinking, "I'll *never* get to sleep tonight"?

- ☐ Toss and turn restlessly in your bed.

- ☐ Take a sleeping pill.

- ☐ Engage in a relaxation exercise.

- ☐ Leave a message on your work supervisor's voice mail that you won't be in tomorrow (call in sick).

- ☐ Drink some alcohol.

- ☐ Other: _____

If you're like most people with insomnia, the previous exercise demonstrates how thoughts, behaviors, and feelings consistent with how you already feel will likely persist. You can liken this process to a CD with a groove etched into it. Once the CD reader gets stuck in this groove, it will continuously play the same broken sound over and over. Nothing will stop this process and get the CD reader out of the groove except an intervention. The intervention is to press a button to skip past the worn area in the CD; without this effort, it would continue indefinitely. Thoughts, behaviors, and feelings can get into a negative groove that requires an intervention to get unstuck. If left to their natural course, thoughts continue to stick in their groove and play the same unwanted sounds over and over. Intervening (or moving the CD reader out of the groove) produces the shift necessary for all three to change.

If your thoughts, behaviors, and feelings can get stuck in a groove in which they're all consistently negative and congruent with each other, what would happen if you were to experience a dramatic shift that produced change in one area? Sure, a check for a million dollars would do the trick, but it's (unfortunately) not a realistic solution. Instead, you might be able to shift to an accepting stance, wherein you accept the fact that you're awake. This accepting stance would make you feel better about being awake. This new perspective would more likely enable you to sleep, because you've shifted away from the anxious distress that interfered with your body's natural sleep-generating system. The shift to an accepting stance would decrease your effort to sleep, which, as we've previously shown, interferes with sleep. Or, suppose that instead of being stuck in the groove of negative thoughts about sleep, you decided to shift your attention to actively dispute these thoughts. Wouldn't you be less upset and better able to sleep? Last, imagine that you decided to conduct an *experiment* to test the idea that you're powerless when you have a night of poor sleep. Imagine that as you collect data on how you function on days after a poor sleep's night, you discover that there's no clear one-to-one correspondence between poor sleep and next-day performance. Wouldn't that discovery alleviate some of the pressure and anxiety to sleep?

These mental exercises demonstrate that what you do, and how you think and feel have consequences for your sleep. The challenge, of course, is how you make these shifts. Is the answer to insomnia to *think positively*? No. It's not that simple. Next let's talk about tools for making the shift.

tools for changing your way of thinking

How do we address thoughts that get in the way of sleeping well? Clearly the answer is not merely thinking positively or, as discussed in the previous chapter, suppressing thoughts, because thought suppression would likely make these thoughts even more pressing. So how do we address thoughts that get in the way of sleeping well? We'll detail a few effective strategies next, including actively challenging thoughts, conducting experiments to test assumptions about sleep, and, in some cases, simply learning more facts about sleep that will dispute inaccurate and sleep-interfering beliefs about sleep.

Myths and Unhelpful Beliefs About Sleep

For each of the following six beliefs, use the scale shown to rate to what extent you believe the belief to be true for you:

Belief	Rating from 0 to 10 (0 = strongly disagree, and 10 = strongly agree)
• If I'm having trouble sleeping, I should try harder.	_____
• If I didn't get sufficient sleep last night, I should try catching up on lost sleep tonight.	_____
• I should sleep at least eight hours every night.	_____
• If I don't sleep well on a given night, I won't be able to cope or adequately function the next day.	_____
• When I'm having a bad night, it's mostly because I didn't sleep well the previous night.	_____
• The consequences of not sleeping well are quite serious.	_____

Some of these beliefs are incorrect, and others might be exaggerated. In some cases these beliefs are rigidly held. Generally, the higher you rate these items, the greater the likelihood that these beliefs will exert a negative influence on your sleep. We'll discuss these beliefs, because they tend to contribute to insomnia or can hinder your progress in enacting some of the behavioral changes we recommended in earlier chapters.

sleep effort and the paradox of insomnia

We already discussed in previous chapters the futility of "trying" to sleep. Can you therefore effectively tell yourself, "Stop trying to sleep"? "What you resist persists" is an oft-used quote attributed to famous psychologist Carl Jung. Have you ever noticed that if you're very focused on avoiding something, you're often unsuccessful at doing so? It seems to be a universal law that if all of your energy is focused on something (such as on avoiding an experience), then you seem to attract the very experience you don't want. In psychology we label this practice *experiential avoidance*. A current movement in psychology is to focus on the importance of "acceptance" rather than on avoidance for overall good mental health, and therapies are available that focus on helping people accept what can't be changed at the moment. The idea is that once there's a shift from denial or from trying harder to solve a problem to true acceptance of the problem and our role in it, new solutions emerge and things tend to improve. Sound crazy? Consider a Chinese finger trap. Have you ever had your finger stuck in one? The instinct is to try to escape by pulling away from the trap. However, as you try to pull your fingers away from each other, you feel the trap tightening, making it even harder to escape. The solution is to do the opposite of your natural instinct; that is, you must willingly accept that you're trapped and relax into it. Push your fingers deeper into the trap, toward each other. This counterintuitive act of relaxing into the trap releases its grip on you.

Like a person whose fingers are trapped in a Chinese finger trap, people with insomnia try hard to fight it. They spend more time in bed trying to increase the window of opportunity for sleep and telling themselves, "Stop thinking and go to sleep!" The natural tendency is to try, try, try, but this tendency to *try*, what we labeled "sleep effort" in chapter 4, tightens the grip of the insomnia trap. If *trying* to sleep is part of the problem, is the answer trying *not* to sleep? There's only one way to find out. Try to stay awake all night tonight while lying in bed in the dark. Don't go to extra efforts to stay awake by drinking coffee, riding your exercise bike, or using your treadmill. Just rest, but stay awake. What do you think will happen? You may say, "But this is what I do every night." But in actuality, what you do each night is try to sleep rather than try *not* to sleep, which is the goal of this experiment. This strategy, called *paradoxical intention*, has been tested and is an oddly effective treatment for difficulties with falling asleep. It's paradoxical because having the intention to *not* sleep has the opposite of its intended effect; that is, it becomes very difficult to stay awake. This *reverse psychology* experiment sounds silly. However, it works because it eliminates the effort to sleep and teaches us that, indeed, sleep occurs most easily when allowed to unfold naturally rather than being forced. An alternative to trying not to sleep is to accept that it's okay if you wake up in the middle of the night. This is, of course, easier said than done, but as you work through your objections, you might find yourself on the other side of the fence. Consider the following examples of acceptance-based thoughts.

Distress-Provoking and Sleep-Interfering Thoughts	Self-Talk with an Accepting Stance
I can't stand this.	It's okay to be awake; it'll pass. I've survived it before.
I've got to do something to get some sleep.	My body will take care of me, so I'll stay out of its way.
I won't be able to function tomorrow.	It might be hard, but I can function okay even when fatigued.
This is terrible; I'm going to take another pill.	I can be at peace while awake during the night.
It seems as if I'll never feel like myself again.	This fatigue will pass; I made this fatalistic prediction because I'm very upset now.

If you still find yourself resisting the accepting stance, read on. We hope that as you learn more, you'll find it more palatable.

beliefs about sleep needs: the golden rule of sleep

One of the first things we learn about sleep comes from our parents. This is the "golden rule of sleep," because it's a very strongly held belief. The golden rule of sleep can be characterized as follows: "Better get a good night's sleep; you have a big day tomorrow." The implicit rule is that good sleep equals good daytime functioning, and poor sleep equals poor daytime functioning. This makes sense, doesn't it? If you slept very little last night, you may not feel at your best the next day. How strongly do you hold onto this golden rule? How flexible are you in this belief?

Following are a couple of beliefs related to the golden rule of sleep. Circle the number that indicates the degree to which you agree or disagree with the following statements:

If I have a good night's sleep, I'll be at my top performance.

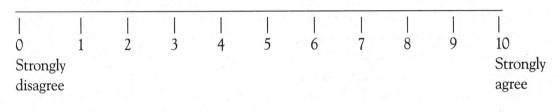

If I have poor sleep tonight, I'll function poorly tomorrow.

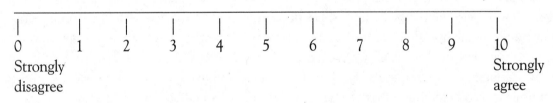

Did you circle these items above 5? Indeed, some days we perform optimally, and other days we perform less optimally or even poorly. Some nights we might sleep better or longer than other nights. Sometimes poor sleep is followed by poor performance, but not always. When we sleep well, it doesn't always translate into optimal performance. Both of these scenarios occur every day and are thus possible, but sometimes people too rigidly hold the belief that poor sleep equals poor functioning 100 percent of the time.

Why does the degree of your belief matter? Consider the strength of Dave's and Helen's beliefs:

Dave's belief: "Generally, I'm more likely to have a better day when I have a good night's sleep, but I do okay either way."

Helen's belief: "If I don't get my eight hours of sleep, I'm useless."

107

Both believe that poor sleep can have a negative impact on their performance. The difference between the two is the degree to which they hold this belief. For Helen sleep is at a premium. She believes she'll be *useless* without adequate sleep, which is a fairly dramatic or extreme view. In contrast, Dave would prefer to have good sleep, yet he expects to function well enough even in the face of poor sleep. Considering only these beliefs, who do you think would more likely cope well with a poor night's sleep? Whose sleep is more likely to be negatively affected by the belief that poor sleep can negatively affect performance? The consequence of Helen's strong belief is increased pressure to sleep. All things being equal, human beings don't sleep well when under pressure, including the pressure to sleep. You can probably see how Helen's strongly held belief increases the chance that she won't sleep well, thus setting the stage for a self-fulfilling prophesy of not functioning well during the day.

Dave's belief incorporates the fact that there are exceptions to the golden rule of sleep. Everyone has experienced exceptions to the golden rule of sleep, such as spending all night awake with someone you are madly in love with and feeling great the next day, or getting good, solid sleep and having a bad day anyway. Remembering that there are exceptions to the rule and that you've managed to cope well with poor sleep in the past will likely reduce the pressure to sleep and reduce performance anxiety around sleep.

Helen completed worksheet 7.1, "Thought Worksheet," every time she was distressed by a sleep-related thought. As she generated and rehearsed alternatives to her rigid belief, the catastrophic prediction that not sleeping well would render her useless dissipated, because it no longer seemed very believable. She also noticed that examining the evidence supporting and disputing her prediction that she would be useless without eight hours of sleep resulted in a more balanced appraisal of this belief, which led to a remarkable reduction in her anxiety and frustration. Reducing Helen's anxiety was important for eliminating the sleep-interfering properties of arousal. It also helped her restrict the time she spent in bed and motivated her to get out of bed when she had difficulty sleeping. Ultimately, after putting all the pieces together, her sleep improved.

Helen's belief that eight hours is the ideal amount of sleep is one of the most common myths concerning sleep. As we learned in chapter 5, the necessary amount of sleep varies among people and changes with age and other circumstances. Some people need much less sleep, and some need much more. People who actually need less sleep than they believe they need find that spending eight hours in bed results in poorer sleep quality compared to spending less time in bed. In addition, believing you *need* eight hours could drive you to go to bed outside of your body clock's window. For example, if you need to rise two hours earlier on a given day and decide to go to bed two hours earlier to allow for eight hours sleep, you may have worse sleep than if you had simply maintained your usual bedtime and shortened your sleep by two hours.

worksheet 7.1 example: Helen's Thought Worksheet

Situation	Mood	Distressing Thoughts or Images	Evidence the Most Distressing Thought Is True	Evidence the Most Distressing Thought May Not Be True	Balanced Alternative Thoughts	Current Mood Rating
Describe the situation in which the distressing thought arose.	*Describe mood in one word and rate its intensity (0–100%).*	*Write any thoughts or images going through your mind. Does the thought activate fears about your well-being or how others may view you?*	*Circle the most distressing thought in the previous column. Write factual evidence for this distressing thought. Stay away from evidence that's not factual; for example, a thought that "feels" true is not factually true.*	*Write evidence that does not support this thought (have you had experiences showing that this thought isn't always true?).*	*Write a thought that better summarizes the evidence for the distressing thought.*	*Copy your feelings from column 2 and rerate their intensity.*
Sitting on the couch alone, close to bedtime	Upset and anxious 90%	If I don't get my 8 hours of sleep, I'm useless.	I feel terrible after a bad night, so I might not be able to do my work.	I don't even know whether I'll get good sleep tonight.	Despite feeling bad at work, I do a good job 99.9% of the time.	Upset and anxious 50%
	Angry 80%	If I'm useless, I'll never be able to function at my meeting.	There was this one time when I got caught laying my head down on my desk.	I'm well-prepared for the meeting.	I've been to dozens of meetings after a bad night, and nothing bad ever happens.	Angry 40%

109

Situation	Mood	Distressing Thoughts or Images	Evidence the Most Distressing Thought Is True	Evidence the Most Distressing Thought May Not Be True	Balanced Alternative Thoughts	Current Mood Rating
		I'm going to look unprepared at my meeting.	It's hard to concentrate after a bad night.	Sometimes I get 8 hours of sleep and still am not at my best.	Predicting poor sleep may increase my chances of sleeping poorly.	
		I can see a humiliating image of me at my meeting.		I can usually "pull it together" for a meeting.	I would never tell someone I love, "You better get 8 hours of sleep or you'll be useless," because I know this wouldn't be helpful.	
		I see myself tossing and turning in bed.		I get good performance reviews at work even though I have insomnia.		

beliefs about your ability to manage poor sleep

At the core of many people's beliefs about insomnia is the fear that they simply can't cope with sleep loss. Actually, most people with insomnia cope reasonably well with sleep loss. Research tells us that despite having to exert extra mental energy, people with insomnia function as well as good sleepers at mental tasks (Bonnet 2005), which suggests that despite feeling lousy, people with insomnia can manage the day's mental demands fairly well. Hyperarousal might explain this surprising finding. The brain seems to compensate for sleep loss with increased activity or resources (producing increased arousal, or hyperarousal), allowing people with insomnia to paradoxically function well during the day.

The unhelpful belief that you can't cope with poor or insufficient sleep can also lead to behaviors that make the insomnia worse. We already discussed some of these behaviors. Now let's turn our attention to what we call *safety behaviors*. Many people with insomnia start reorganizing their lives to protect themselves from the predicted negative consequences of poor sleep. These changes are aimed at making them feel safer from the consequences of sleep loss. Playing it safe can be a good strategy for making some choices in life, yet being strongly driven by safety can go too far, particularly when it's done to cope with a problem. Indeed this habit can unintentionally contribute to the very problem it intends to diminish. People living with conditions such as insomnia, anxiety, and chronic pain are prone to overuse the play-it-safe strategy. They may cancel appointments and spend the day resting in response to insufficient sleep, fears, and pain, which are examples of safety behaviors. Unfortunately safety behaviors end up worsening or preventing recovery from the condition they're intended to relieve. Here's an example:

> *Paul suffers from chronic low-back pain and has noticed that when he sleeps poorly, his pain is worse during the day. So, after a bad night, he calls in sick, cancels social plans, and tries to rest as much as possible. Avoiding activities during the day makes him feel safe. After all, it minimizes the probability of making a bad move or having to sit for a long time, which can worsen his back pain. However, avoidance is a double-edged sword. The flip side is that by being more sedentary, Paul weakens his muscles, consequently becoming more vulnerable to injuries, aches, and pains. Moreover, as he keeps calling in sick each time he has a bad night, Paul starts to worry at night that if he doesn't sleep, he'll miss work and need to cancel activities he usually enjoys, such as social events. Worrying will intensify his desperation for sleep, increase his sleep effort, and make sleep even more elusive. Paul's safety behaviors also obscure the fact that he has seen past evidence that he'll most likely be okay at work even after a poor night's sleep. He has gone to work before and experienced no catastrophic consequences. So, avoiding going to work and cancelling social appointments actually sustains Paul's pain and insomnia.*

Complete the following checklist to see the extent to which you engage in insomnia-specific safety behaviors.

Safety Behavior Checklist

People with insomnia tend to engage in a variety of safety behaviors. Do you recognize any of these?

☐ Canceling appointments after a poor night's sleep

☐ Trying to suppress or avoid certain thoughts

☐ Trying to keep images from appearing in your mind as you try to sleep

☐ Drinking alcohol when something upsetting comes to mind

☐ Taking a sleeping pill if you notice tension or physical sensations associated with being unable to sleep

☐ Avoiding interacting with people after a poor night's sleep

☐ Engaging in any behavior aimed at reducing an unpleasant thought or feeling related to insomnia

Engaging in safety behaviors, such as canceling activities after a poor night's sleep, may have three adverse effects: First, it confirms for you the idea that you can't manage the negative effects of insomnia. The belief that you can't cope with insomnia increases your emotional distress when you have difficulty falling asleep at night. The distress, which is an alertness-promoting factor, also increases the probability that you'll have difficulty sleeping at night. The second adverse effect of a safety behavior is that it prevents you from experiencing evidence that might contradict your belief. For example, Paul's avoidance of activities prevented him from potentially having an enjoyable day. Likewise, if you're afraid something negative will happen during the day because of your insomnia, avoiding activities and obligations would prevent you from learning that on the overwhelming majority of days, the things you fear most don't actually happen. The third adverse effect is that canceling activities after experiencing poor sleep reinforces the belief that sleeping poorly is harmful. For example, when you cancel a fun activity, you feel sorry you have to miss it. As a result, you have evidence, as flawed as it is, that poor sleep has significant deleterious consequences, because it prevents you from doing things you like to do.

Generally, safety behaviors promote the notion that you can't manage the negative effects of insomnia and preclude the opportunity to gather evidence that might be inconsistent with this notion. The conclusion is to avoid *avoidance*! Here are the steps for dealing with safety behaviors:

1. The first step is to identify any safety behaviors you have. Start with the "Safety Behavior Checklist," and think through your own situation to identify safety behaviors that aren't listed.

2.   Next, challenge the beliefs underlying the safety behaviors you've identified.

3.   The third step is to stop engaging in the safety behaviors.

In some cases you might need to design a small experiment to test a belief underlying one of your safety behaviors. For example, if one of the safety behaviors you identified (step 1) is the tendency to call in sick after a difficult night, one possible underlying belief (step 2) is that you won't be able to handle a full workload unless you sleep well enough. Following is a possible experiment that can help you test this assertion (step 3).

First track how you felt on a day you called in sick because you didn't sleep well. Then track how you felt on a day you were tempted to call in sick but, for the sake of the experiment, didn't. Compare these two days. Can you identify drawbacks to canceling activities? For example, do you now have even more on your plate because you didn't accomplish what you had planned? Do you have to make up for the lost work now, on top of your busy schedule? Does a coworker get upset when you don't show up at work? Most people report that they felt much better when they stuck to their regular activities and didn't cancel any.

People use safety behaviors because they produce a positive short-term benefit, such as reduced anxiety. However, in retrospect people also often find more negative than positive long-term consequences to engaging in safety behaviors. Last, there's reason to believe that avoidance may worsen whatever other conditions you're dealing with. Safety behaviors have been implicated in contributing to:

- Chronic pain: Avoiding activities for fear of injury results in secondary pain from underuse (Philips 1987).

- Depression: Avoiding people has the long-term consequence of social isolation and decreased exposure to potentially enjoyable things, thus making you even more depressed (Lewinsohn and Libet 1972).

- Anxiety: Avoiding anxiety-provoking situations for fear of experiencing anxiety sensations strengthens anxiety and increases the likelihood of experiencing more anxiety in a future similar situation (Salkovskis 1991).

Look for opportunities to challenge beliefs that underlie your safety behaviors, and pay careful attention to the evidence for good coping that already exists in your life.

when everything is about sleep

One year Brian's dog brought fleas into the house. The bites itched, and Brian spent a lot of time bathing the dog, and vacuuming and spraying the house. The fleas continued to hang around, so he tried to catch them, most often catching them as they bit because he could feel the sting of the bite, look down, and grab the flea. Brian became so aware of the fleas that he began seeing them before they had a chance to bite. He was always on the lookout for a flea and became pretty good at catching them. While this strategy was initially pretty effective, he was so focused on the fleas that every sensation on his skin seemed like a flea (even though there wasn't always a flea there when he looked). However every twenty times or so, he was correct, and there was a flea he could catch. Brian was miserable; his focus on the fleas drove him crazy. He constantly felt bugs crawling on his skin or saw them in the periphery even though they weren't always there. He began misinterpreting normal sensations on his skin as fleas. Brian was a rational man and was bothered by this odd sensory illusion. He noticed that he had become so upset by these unwelcome visitors that he focused all of his attention on them in order to catch them. I (C. E. C.) suggested that he try to divert his attention away from the fleas to see if this misperception continued. He decided to focus on alternative explanations for the creepy-crawly sensations on his skin. For example, the weather had abruptly become cold, and the heater was on almost constantly. Brian noticed that his skin had become very dry, and dry skin gets itchy. This revelation (and a few persistent flea dips for his dog) resolved the preoccupation with the fleas and the misperception of creepy crawlies on his skin.

Did Brian's flea problem help him understand his insomnia? Strangely, yes! Brian learned that when people become upset, they often focus increasingly *more* attention on the problem. While this makes sense, people can focus so much on the problem that it actually adds to the problem. We know that people with insomnia are more focused on things that relate to sleep than people without insomnia (Espie et al. 2006). Why would this matter? People with insomnia are, in a sense, constantly looking for fleas and sometimes finding fleas where there are none; that is, they're always scanning for information in the environment that confirms that they won't be able to sleep or function after poor sleep. If they look hard enough, they'll find such threats, real or imagined, just as in Brian's experience with the fleas. This means that if you're concerned that poor sleep will lead to fatigue, you'll perceive fatigue more readily than someone who's less focused on it. Try the following exercise.

Rate your current state of well-being:

Terrible								Great
0	1	2	3	4	5	6	7	8

Spend five minutes directing your attention to how you feel. Do your legs hurt? Do your eyes feel heavy? Are your muscles sore? If so, where? Your neck, shoulders, head, back? Are your eyes tired? Do they burn? Continue to focus on how you feel for five minutes. Don't read on until you're done.

After the five minutes of monitoring have passed, rate how you feel:

Terrible								Great
0	1	2	3	4	5	6	7	8

Now spend five minutes directing your attention outward. Take note of your surroundings. Notice the colors, patterns, textures, sounds, and smells. Spend all five minutes noticing with open curiosity all that's around you. After five minutes have elapsed, rate how you feel now:

Terrible   Great

0   1   2   3   4   5   6   7   8

Reflect on what you experienced under each condition. Most people find that focusing inward worsens how they feel. Focusing on things other than how you feel can be a very effective tool in coping with sleep loss. If you focus your attention on the tasks of the day, you'll likely experience less fatigue than if you woke up and monitored your fatigue experience throughout the day.

the sleep scapegoat

Focusing on your internal state might also make you more likely to attribute any ill feelings to insufficient sleep, even when there may be other (more accurate) explanations for them. Just as Brian often mistakenly attributed his itchy sensations to fleas biting, a person with insomnia who's focused on fatigue, negative mood, or concentration problems tends to attribute these to poor sleep, ignoring alternative explanations for fatigue-related symptoms. Even doctors might make the mistake of assuming that fatigue is always related to sleep. Possible alternative explanations for fatigue include:

- Taking medications with fatigue or drowsiness as a side effect (for example, antihistamines)

- Boredom or low stimulation

- Dehydration

- Caffeine rebound (while the body breaks down caffeine, one of its withdrawal symptoms is fatigue)

- Spending too much time in bed

- Negative mood

- Diet

- Chronic stress

- Depression

- Pain

- Anxiety

- Inactivity

- Overactivity or physical exertion

- Lack of physical conditioning, excess weight, or both

- Cardiovascular disease

- Eye strain

- Constipation

- Low iron levels (anemia)

- Candida

- Infections

- Medical conditions, such as hypothyroidism

- Post-lunch dip in body temperature

- Others: _____

As you can see, it's a pretty long list and it's not even exhaustive. Clearly, there are many, many other explanations than poor sleep for feeling fatigue. Most of these are self-evident; however, the relationship between fatigue and the post-lunch dip in body temperature may require more elaboration. For most people who sleep at night and are awake during the day, there's a natural, very small dip in core body temperature usually between 1:00 and 3:00 p.m. This dip in temperature involves a temporary decrease in the alertness signal and an increase in fatigue that can make it more difficult to concentrate. Some people explain this experience by attributing it to a heavy lunch. While overeating can produce some lethargy, a daily afternoon experience of mild, transient fatigue is most likely due to the dip in body temperature. This is a very common time for people to take a coffee break, perhaps to compensate for this natural dip in energy level. Unfortunately, drinking coffee at this time may do little to improve this transient fatigue. If the fatigue dissipates, it may have more to do with the fact that the temperature dip is temporary and passes naturally even without caffeine. If you do consume caffeine, your body will experience rebound fatigue several hours later because of caffeine withdrawal. So consuming caffeine to cope with a natural and transient dip in energy is an ineffective strategy that backfires because caffeine withdrawal later increases fatigue. You're probably more likely to reach for a cup of coffee if you tend to automatically (and incorrectly) attribute the dip in energy to poor sleep at night. This illustrates an important point: the more attentive or focused you are on your lack of sleep and its potential negative consequences, the more likely you are to be caught in a self-perpetuating cycle whereby overfocusing on threats to sleep leads to actual worsening of sleep.

what is sleep misperception?

Brian *felt* fleas that weren't there; does this mean he was crazy? Absolutely not! When we're overfocused on one thing, particularly if it's something upsetting or distressing, we're prone to misperceive sensations. People with insomnia feel more alert when in bed and may be more likely to mislabel periods of sleep as periods of wakefulness. In other words, they can misperceive being asleep as being awake. One possible explanation for this misperception is that people with insomnia are hyperalert. As we previously described, the brains of people with insomnia are hyperactive in areas that should be less active when falling asleep. This hyperactivity may lead people to misperceive natural and common mini-awakenings as a block of wakefulness. In contrast, people without insomnia are more likely to perceive these very same mini-awakenings as sleep, disregarding the brief interruptions in sleep. Another reason for sleep misperception among people with insomnia is related to memory. Because memories experienced during sleep aren't accessible during waking hours, people who don't have prolonged awakenings don't remember the brief awakenings and, in the morning, perceive their sleep as uninterrupted. In contrast, people with insomnia who experience longer periods of wakefulness at night may form memories during nighttime wakefulness that they can access in the morning. Therefore they assume that if they remember large parts of the night, they must have been awake the entire time. In reality they likely had multiple periods of sleep that they don't remember.

> *Chris suffered from chronic anxiety and, when describing her sleep problem, stated, "I don't sleep." Actually, it's unlikely that she doesn't sleep. While it's possible to have some nights without any sleep at all, this is very rare. People always produce some sleep; they just sleep less when they have insomnia. I (C. E. C.) asked Chris how much sleep she usually got on average, and she answered, "None." A review of her sleep logs revealed "0" in every column. I asked her what she did while in bed for the seven and a half hours each night, and she answered that she rested. She explained that she lay in bed with the lights out and television off for seven and a half hours, and was sure that she never slept. Later in our conversation she complained that her husband had mentioned her snoring, which bothered her, because she knew she wasn't sleeping. She also complained of having had a bad dream one night even though she had recorded no sleep. I asked her to wear a sensitive motion detector on her wrist, which records movement throughout the night and can estimate how much sleep a person gets. The following week we looked at the recording from the device. She was irritated that it recorded almost six hours of sleep each night, and complained that the device couldn't be right. I invited her to spend the night in our sleep laboratory, and a recording of her brain activity at night revealed that she slept for seven hours. She still insisted she hadn't slept at all.*

While Chris is an extreme case, many studies show that some people with insomnia underestimate how long they sleep and overestimate the amount of time they spend awake at night. What problems could misperception cause? Take a moment to ponder this question before proceeding.

Sleep misperception is distressing because it means that the golden rule of sleep is being (seriously) violated. In other words, you're convinced that you're not getting enough sleep, which, in turn, means that you won't be able to function. This conviction naturally provokes anxiety and increases the pressure to produce more sleep. As we previously discussed, high levels of worry and feeling pressured to sleep interfere with sleep. Look at the following statements. Who would you predict would be *more* anxious about sleep?

- Someone who believes he didn't sleep at all

- Someone who believes she slept poorly for six hours

The cost of having the inaccurate belief, "I don't sleep," is anxiety. Anything that provokes anxiety will make sleep even worse. When you think you didn't sleep *at all*, consider the possibility that you might have dozed off into light sleep but, because you were frequently aware of being awake, concluded that you didn't sleep. Do you remember the entire night? If not, why? We remember our days, so why not remember the night in its entirety? If the television was on all night, can you remember every show and every plot line? Why not? Were you startled awake by a noise? If so, this implies you were asleep (however briefly). You may have slept very little, which is better than thinking you didn't sleep at all. If you continue to struggle with sleep misperception, a sleep specialist may be able to help. Some specialists can provide a device like the one I (C. E. C.) gave Chris, which will help you discover hidden sleep. Researchers improved the perception of sleep in volunteers who came to a sleep lab and were awakened each time their brain waves indicated they had slept. After repeated awakenings, the volunteers learned to recognize sleep more readily and accurately (Downey and Bonnet 1992). Although this is not a practical solution to misperceiving sleep, it's an intriguing discovery nonetheless. Being open to the possibility that beliefs and hyperarousal of the brain color your sleep perception and that you're probably getting more sleep than you think can help you improve your sleep, particularly if you also follow our earlier recommendations.

catastrophizing about the consequences of poor sleep

Some people with insomnia become very anxious about the consequences of poor sleep. Usually these worries are blown out of proportion. To help sift through the true and imagined consequences, we recommend that you generate a list of worries about your sleep. Start with the most salient (distressing) worry and ask yourself, "And then what?" until you've taken this worry to its most extreme end. See Helen's example, which follows. Don't censor yourself as you engage in this exercise, even if you know rationally that the worry is probably unrealistic. Fully explore your deepest fears from your less rational moments. You can examine the irrationality of some of these thoughts later.

HELEN'S WORRIES ABOUT SLEEP

1. *If I don't get eight hours, I'll be useless.*
      And *then* what?

2. *I won't be able to get my work done.*
      And *then* what?

3. *I could get into trouble at work.*
      And *then* what?

4. *I would feel humiliated. Plus, I could potentially get fired.*
      And *then* what?

5. *I wouldn't be able to pay my bills.*
      And *then* what?

6. *I could get evicted.*
      And *then* what?

7. *I could wind up homeless.*
      And *then* what?

MY WORRIES ABOUT SLEEP

1. _____
      And *then* what?

2. _____
      And *then* what?

3. _____
      And *then* what?

4. _____
      And *then* what?

5. _____
      And *then* what?

6. _____
      And *then* what?

7. _____
      And *then* what?

Many people are quite surprised when they see their hidden fears in writing. It's not uncommon to discover a fear of going crazy, of having serious physical illness and disability, and even of winding up homeless, which are terrifying possibilities. With so much on the line (for example, a threat of illness, insanity, or homelessness), it's no wonder that you experience performance anxiety about sleep every night. We ask people to do this exercise to help them explore pressures to sleep that are perhaps hidden from awareness. We call these beliefs *catastrophizing*, because they focus on the most unlikely, worst-possible imagined outcome. Since the catastrophic predictions are threatening and since humans don't sleep well under pressure and threats, the cost of having such beliefs is increased insomnia. Now let's turn our attention to the rationality or accuracy of these beliefs. How likely do any of these possibilities seem to you? How often would insomnia underlie homelessness, physical disability, or mental illness? Is this catastrophizing? One helpful way to determine whether you may be catastrophizing is to ask yourself, "If someone I loved had this thought, would I be likely to think it's accurate?" In other words, if someone expressed a fear of becoming homeless, would you think it was a likely outcome of insomnia? Probably not! If such inaccurate thoughts are so detrimental to sleep, they're worthy of direct challenge. If you have sleep-related worries, it's important to remind yourself that there have been thousands of instances in your life when you've coped well with sleep disturbance, and probably little to no instances in which a catastrophic event occurred. Allowing these beliefs to lurk unexplored beneath the surface of your awareness increases their sleep-interfering power. Instead, expose these beliefs to the light, because examining and challenging such beliefs will alleviate some of the self-imposed pressure to sleep. You may find it helpful to use worksheet 7.1, "Thought Worksheet" (at the end of this chapter) to challenge catastrophic thoughts or any other distressing sleep-related thought.

other myths about sleep

One of the final and most basic ways to change your thinking is simply to have access to correct information about sleep. For some people, reading about sleep and proper sleep practices is enough to produce change. Following are some common myths (Morin 1993) and why they're either not true or, at the very least, less true than most people with insomnia think. In addition, the last column provides one example of why it's harmful to strongly believe these myths.

MYTHS ABOUT SLEEP AND WHY THEY'RE NOT HELPFUL

Myth	Why It's Not True	Consequence of Believing This Myth
"I absolutely require eight hours of sleep to function during the day."	There's a wide range of sleep needs. The average amount of sleep needed for an adult is unknown but is probably less than eight hours. Second, sleep duration is only one of many determinants of daytime functioning; within reason, sleep quality is probably more important than the total amount of sleep.	Eight hours becomes a magical number that creates anxiety if it's not reached. It may be an unrealistic number for you (and for most adults).
"If I've had good sleep, I should wake up feeling refreshed."	After waking, it's natural to spend up to thirty minutes feeling groggy. This is called sleep inertia or sleep drunkenness, which is transient and is likely affected by the sleep stage from which you were awakened. If you are a night person, you may experience more sleep inertia than the average person.	This belief can become a self-fulfilling prophecy. If you awaken and think, "I feel terrible; I'll never be able to get through the day," chances are you'll have a more difficult time and sleep performance anxiety will increase, leading to worse sleep.
"I wake up a couple of times each night. Even though I fall back to sleep pretty quickly, I know it must be having a negative effect."	Brief arousals are a normal part of the sleep process. Although most are not long enough to be remembered in the morning, the average number of awakenings per night is twelve (Bonnet and Arand 2007). A normal amount of time to spend awake in bed is up to thirty minutes.	Believing that you should never wake up during the night, even if you fall back to sleep right away, is unrealistic and will only produce anxiety. The anxiety may eventually produce more-serious insomnia.
"If I spend more time in bed, I'll get more sleep and feel better the next day."	Sleep quality is more important than quantity. In addition to interfering with the sleep driver and your biological clock, spending extra time in bed may increase depression.	This conviction may worsen your sleep and mood. A weakened sleep driver compensates for increased time in bed by decreasing the drive for sleep.

121

Myth	Why It's Not True	Consequence of Believing This Myth
"I'm older, so insomnia is just a fact of life."	While there are increased awakenings from sleep with aging, not all older adults develop insomnia. There are also things you can do (as outlined in this book) to prevent insomnia as you age.	You may neglect to make changes that could improve your sleep.
"I can't do anything to help my sleep because insomnia is caused by a chemical imbalance."	There's no evidence of this, and sleeping pills don't target a chemical imbalance.	This myth sends you the message that you have no power to affect your sleep. A loss of confidence in your ability to sleep further undermines your sleep.

taking action

1. Complete worksheet 7.1, "Thought Worksheet," when you experience a distressing thought related to sleep.

2. Did you check off any safety behaviors on the "Safety Behavior Checklist" (earlier in this chapter)? If so, devise an experiment using worksheet 7.2, "Changing Safety Behaviors."

3. Complete worksheet 7.3, "Alternative Reasons for Fatigue," when you're distressed by daytime fatigue or fatigue-related symptoms such as poor concentration, inattention, or negative mood.

4. Monitor your sleep on a sleep log.

5. Most important, continue with other sleep recommendations from earlier chapters, such as getting out of bed when you can't sleep and restricting your time in bed to more accurately match the amount of sleep your body is currently producing.

worksheet 7.1: Thought Worksheet

Complete this worksheet whenever you experience a distressing sleep-related thought.

Situation	Mood	Distressing Thoughts or Images	Evidence the Most Distressing Thought Is True	Evidence the Most Distressing Thought May Not Be True	Balanced Alternative Thoughts	Current Mood Rating
Describe the situation in which the distress-ing thought arose.	*Describe mood in one word and rate its intensity (0–100%).*	*Write any thoughts or images going through your mind. Does the thought activate fears about your well-being or how others may view you?*	*Circle the most distressing thought in the previous column. Write factual evidence for this distressing thought. Stay away from evidence that's not factual; for example, a thought that "feels" true is not factually true.*	*Write evidence that does not support this thought (have you had experiences showing that this thought isn't always true?).*	*Write a thought that better summarizes the evidence for the distressing thought.*	*Copy your feelings from column 2 and rerate their intensity.*

worksheet 7.2: Changing Safety Behaviors

Safety Behavior	What Message Are You Sending Yourself by Engaging in This Behavior?	What Will You Do to Show That It's Not True?	Result of the Experiment
Example: I take a sleeping pill in the middle of the night when I notice I'm worked up.	It sends a message that I've lost all confidence in my ability to sleep. It also says that I don't think I can cope with feeling worked up.	I'll refrain from taking the pill in the middle of the night and see what happens.	I felt better during the day and less groggy on the days I didn't take the pill. Even though it was initially frightening not to take the pill, I noticed that if I took the pill, I tended to fall back to sleep only a few minutes sooner than on the nights when I just waited it out.
1.			
2.			
3.			
4.			

worksheet 7.3: Alternative Reasons for Fatigue

Rate the probability that the following reasons account for some of your fatigue.

Likelihood 0–100%	Reasons for Fatigue
	Taking medications that have fatigue or drowsiness as a side effect
	Boredom or low stimulation
	Dehydration
	Caffeine rebound
	Spending too much time in bed
	Negative mood
	Diet
	Chronic stress
	Depression
	Pain
	Anxiety
	Inactivity
	Overactivity or physical exertion
	Lack of physical conditioning, excess weight, or both
	Cardiovascular disease
	Eye strain
	Constipation
	Low iron levels (anemia)
	Candida
	Infections
	Medical conditions, such as hypothyroidism
	Post-lunch dip in body temperature
	Other reasons: _____

summing up

- Your beliefs about sleep may worsen your insomnia. Changing your beliefs can increase your confidence in your ability to sleep, and reduce the severity of your insomnia and the amount of time you lie awake in bed.

- Changing your beliefs isn't easy, because they can be ingrained.

- The most harmful beliefs are:

    You need to apply effort to sleep or to compensate for sleep loss.

    A specific amount of sleep is needed.

    You can't cope or adequately function when you have insomnia.

    Feeling bad during the day is always from lack of sleep.

    Something *terrible* will happen to you as a result of insomnia.

- Strategies for change include:

    Learning about sleep myths

    Actively challenging unhelpful beliefs

    Testing assumptions about sleep by conducting an experiment

    Decreasing safety behaviors

    Moving toward acceptance

issues with substances and medications

In previous chapters we discussed the essentials of effective insomnia treatment that apply to the vast majority of people with insomnia. We emphasized the importance of keeping wakeful activities and wakefulness out of the bedroom, maintaining a regular schedule, and matching the amount of time you spend in bed to how much sleep your body currently produces. We also addressed the beliefs that get in the way of your sleep, and introduced methods for calming an overactive mind. In this chapter we address the effects of certain substances on sleep, including caffeine, nicotine, and alcohol. Consumption of some of these substances in excess or at the wrong time of day may interfere with your sleep and consequently prevent full recovery from your insomnia, even if you implement the essential components of treatment discussed earlier. Many of the commonsense recommendations regarding substances will seem familiar. You may have already tried following them without experiencing marked improvement in your sleep. One thing to consider is that changing your consumption of substances with proven negative effects on sleep is necessary but not sufficient for improving your sleep. For maximum benefit, put this into action along with the other pieces of the treatment. We also briefly discuss the effects of sleep medications on sleep. We conclude with a discussion of what effects medications you might be taking for depression, anxiety, or pain might have on your sleep. We encourage you to continue taking medications your doctor prescribed for these conditions, because they're likely essential for your treatment of these conditions and many will likely benefit your sleep as well.

---

alertness-promoting factors

Caffeine: It's common for those who are struggling with daytime fatigue to use caffeine in an attempt to increase their alertness. However, caffeine is a stimulant, and stimulants interfere with sleep. People differ in their sensitivity to the effects of caffeine, partly because the time required for the body to eliminate half the total amount of caffeine, known as its "half-life," depends on how well your liver functions, your age, and what other medications you're taking. On average, caffeine's half-life in adults is approximately four hours. Also of note, oral contraceptives and pregnancy increase sensitivity to caffeine, and smoking decreases it. Caffeine's effects on the body also vary with your body size and your individual level of sensitivity to its effects. Therefore, it's difficult to determine the amount and timing of caffeine consumption that would interfere with the sleep of any given person.

We know that caffeine can disrupt sleep long after its alerting effects are felt. Caffeine can prolong the time it takes to fall asleep and lead to light or restless sleep. Caffeine is believed to block the effects of the sleep driver, which, as mentioned earlier, helps regulate sleep. Caffeine can also worsen preexisting problems, such as heartburn or ulcers, which can further disrupt sleep. Caffeine is found in many sources, including chocolate (particularly the very dark variety that's gaining popularity), teas, many soft drinks, and some over-the-counter medications, such as cold medications and diet pills. Compounding the problem is the difficulty discerning the amount of caffeine in some of these substances. For example, the amount of caffeine in coffee and tea depends on their preparation. However, there's no reason to necessarily give up your morning cup of coffee. A good rule of thumb is to aim for less than 250 milligrams of caffeine each day (an average mug of coffee has just over half this amount), and never consume caffeine within six hours of your bedtime. Keep in mind that some people are particularly sensitive to the effects of caffeine and should therefore avoid it past lunchtime. When you evaluate caffeine's impact on you, it's also important to consider its side effects.

Caffeine can cause heart palpitations, anxiety, and restlessness. Caffeine is a double-edged sword, because it can also produce rebound symptoms, such as fatigue, difficulty concentrating, and headaches. Because insomnia also causes these symptoms, it's difficult to discern their cause in a person with insomnia who consumes large amounts of caffeine. Some people neglect to consider the possibility that caffeine use might be causing their fatigue or irritability, and instead attribute these symptoms only to poor sleep. This attribution bias could further increase their distress about insomnia and contribute to worse sleep at night, an unfortunate unintended consequence. Some people with insomnia report that simply reducing their caffeine consumption made them feel better during the day, probably due to the elimination of the symptoms of a caffeine crash.

Cigarettes: Cigarette smoking is also incompatible with sleep. Cigarettes contain nicotine, which is a stimulant. Some people are surprised to hear this and say that cigarettes are relaxing, which is not exactly accurate. When the body breaks down nicotine, withdrawal symptoms, such as agitation and tension, result. Smoking another cigarette adds nicotine to the bloodstream, reducing the tension and agitation produced by withdrawal from the previous cigarette. The smoker experiences this process as relaxing. In reality, rather than relaxing tension from everyday stresses, a cigarette only treats the tension and agitation that resulted from withdrawal from the previous cigarette. Because there are many health reasons to quit smoking, we would like to encourage you to quit. It's important to be prepared for a few poor nights of sleep as you go through the withdrawal process, because one symptom of quitting the habit of smoking cigarettes is sleeplessness, which can last several weeks. If you expect some degree of temporary sleep disruption, you'll be able to discount it for what it is. Quitting smoking isn't easy, but using multiple strategies can increase the odds of success. For example, a combination of medical help (nicotine patches or gums and medications) and psychological help (psychotherapy or a support group) increase the likelihood of success (Clinical Practice Guideline Treating Tobacco Use and Dependence 2008 Update Panel, Liaisons, and Staff 2008).

the paradoxical effects of alcohol

People with insomnia may attempt to medicate their sleep problem with alcohol, because it can have an immediately calming effect and hasten the onset of sleep in people without alcoholism. Using alcohol to help with sleep is fairly common among people with insomnia. However, while it's sometimes helpful at the beginning of the night, alcohol leads to shallow and disrupted sleep later in the night, because the body breaks it down rapidly so that little alcohol is left in the blood in the middle of the night. Symptoms of withdrawal from excessive alcohol use are well known and are colloquially termed "hangover." It's less known that even a small amount of alcohol close to bedtime can lead to withdrawal symptoms in the middle of the night, albeit they're less dramatic than a hangover. The most common middle-of-the-night symptom is shallow sleep with multiple awakenings. Also, because alcohol decreases REM sleep during the first half of the night, vivid dreams and even nightmares might emerge during the second half of the night. This phenomenon is known as *REM rebound*, which is a significant increase in REM sleep following its suppression earlier in the night. While some people believe that REM sleep is a deep stage of sleep, in fact it's a stage of sleep that more closely resembles wakeful brain activity than deep-sleep activity. Sweating may be another alcohol withdrawal symptom during the second half of the night. Alcohol consumption close to bedtime could also lead to greater collapse in the upper airways, leading to snoring and worsening of sleep apnea, which ultimately result in poorer quality of sleep. Thus, a costly loss of quality sleep replaces alcohol's immediate benefits. One final drawback may be that over time, larger and larger quantities of alcohol will be necessary to produce the same effect, so insomnia may prompt alcohol abuse (Ford and Kamerow 1989). Alcoholism involves poor sleep, characterized by prolonged time to fall asleep, multiple awakenings, and decreased slow-wave sleep and REM sleep (Vitiello 1997; Weissman et al. 1997; Foster and Peters 1999; Roehrs and Roth 2001) Unfortunately the sleep disturbances in alcoholics can persist for months and even years after they've quit drinking (Adamson and Burdick 1973; Drummond et al. 1998).

sleep medications

Ned came into my (C. E. C.) clinic and sheepishly admitted that when I had explained the behavioral insomnia treatment to him a few years ago, it sounded too hard, so he asked the psychiatrist who'd referred him to me to prescribe a new sleep medication. He explained that he used to take a sleeping pill that was very effective but had stopped working, which was the reason his doctor had referred him to my clinic. The new medication worked well for the first few months and then gradually lost its effectiveness, just as the old sleep medication had done. He was then switched to a different pill with much the same result. Frustration with having to constantly switch medications triggered Ned's return to my clinic.

Ned's story isn't that unusual. Some sleep medications lose their effectiveness over time. As the body builds up tolerance, a higher dose is required. However, because higher and higher doses might lead to unwanted and dangerous side effects, a switch to another medication is often recommended. The emotional roller coaster of medications working and then not working is frustrating and prompts some to seek approaches to treating their insomnia that don't involve use of medication.

Traditional Prescribed Sleep Medications

Not all medications prescribed by your doctor for sleep are classified as sleep medications by the U.S. Food and Drug Administration (FDA). In this section we discuss FDA-approved sleep medications only. Sleep medications provide a quick, easy, and effective short-term solution to insomnia for some people. Others may experience no benefits, and yet others may conclude that the negative side effects are unacceptable even if the medication helps them sleep better. One side effect that has garnered attention in the past few years led to an FDA warning in 2007. The FDA warned that some popular sleep medications involve doing things in your sleep that you may not remember (FDA 2007). News media covered stories on instances in which people engaged in sleepwalking and other unwanted or unsafe activities, such as eating in the middle of the night without awareness and driving a motor vehicle in the middle of the night without remembering a thing in the morning. Though these cases are rare, they received high publicity and, in the minds of many people with insomnia, raised concerns about the use of sleeping pills. Always discuss with a doctor the pros and cons of taking particular sleep medications.

We also caution against stopping sleep medications abruptly, because doing so can cause poor sleep, known as *rebound insomnia* (Greenblatt 1992). Likely a withdrawal symptom, the disrupted sleep doesn't necessarily reflect the underlying sleep problem. The rebound insomnia is often falsely interpreted as evidence: "I can't sleep without sleep medication." This creates a psychological dependence on the medication, making it even harder to get off it. If you and your doctor decide it's time to get off the medication, it's best to do so gradually and be willing to tolerate a few nights of less-than-optimal sleep.

Research shows that people who use sleep medications can benefit from the type of treatment in this book (Verbeek, Schreuder, and Declerck 1999), so there's no reason to stop. However, if you're using a sleep medication, you might need to modify some of our recommendations. For example, because some sleep medications are long acting, you'll need to consult your doctor before restricting your time in bed, as recommended in chapter 5. If you continue to take prescribed long-acting sleep medication while following the treatment in this book, when you first wake up, you might not be able to judge how well you slept because the long-acting sleep medications have a carryover effect that make you feel less than optimally alert on waking.

Also be aware of the potential impact of taking sleep medication on your level of commitment to the CBT described in this book. Many people with insomnia lose confidence in their ability to sleep, believing that sleep is out of their control. This is a very frightening prospect, given that sleep is a basic and very necessary human function. Taking a sleeping pill that works alleviates this anxiety because you might reason, " At least there's *something* I can do to help my sleep problem." The flip side is that taking sleep medication reinforces the idea that something's terribly wrong with your ability to sleep. In that way, taking sleeping pills can further undermine your confidence in your ability to sleep and cope. Holding this belief may make you less likely to make some of the more difficult changes in your sleep behaviors that we recommend in this book. If you're taking sleep medications but still have sleep problems, the treatment discussed in this book may still help you improve your sleep and will allow you to regain your trust in your body's ability to produce sleep. Since you haven't slept well on medication and your sleep will likely improve without changing medications, it will show you that there's something within your power to help you sleep better. If your ultimate goal is to get off sleep medications but you don't yet feel ready to do so, you might be in a better position to make this decision after you learn what you can do to help yourself sleep better. When you're ready to get off the sleep medication, consult with your doctor about tapering off of it.

If you've used sleep medication for a while and are ambivalent about it, you may try to fall asleep without the medication and resort to taking it when you've given up trying to fall asleep. This is not the best way to take sleep medication long term, because it promotes psychological dependence, which is exactly what you fear. If you've taken a sleeping medication for a while, it's best to take it at bedtime on a regular schedule. For example, if you take sleeping pills an average of four times a week, decide which four nights you'll take them, and take them at bedtime. In particular, if you take a pill every night, it's best to continue taking it every night at bedtime rather than first waiting to see if you can fall asleep without it. This achieves two goals: it reduces psychological dependence and removes the question, "Should I take a pill tonight?" which inevitably increases sleep anxiety and interferes with sleep.

antihistamines

Some over-the-counter medications have FDA approval for use as sleep aids. The active ingredients in these medications are usually diphenhydramine (for example, in Benadryl) or doxylamine (found in many cold medications). These medications work by blocking the effects of an alertness-promoting chemical in the brain called "histamine," hence their name "antihistamines." Antihistamines can be effective for some people, particularly with mild insomnia (Morin et al. 2005), but they may also produce a "hangover effect" (Mendelson et al. 2004). Whenever you have a hangover effect in the morning, there's a risk misattributing it to poor sleep, but doing so may increase anxiety and sleep effort, which may exacerbate the insomnia. As with prescription sleep medications, there's also a risk of tolerance and psychological dependence.

over-the-counter or herbal sleep remedies

So-called "natural" medications, such as herbal compounds or dietary supplements, have become a big business. Some people consider them more benign than compounds sold by large drug companies. However, these medications aren't regulated, so there's no way of knowing whether you're getting the stated dose in each capsule. Two natural sleep remedies that have been studied are the herb valerian and the hormone melatonin. Valerian seems to provide some modest sleep benefits (Schulz, Stolz, and Müller 1994), but it does have side effects, including morning hangover and headache. Evidence for the efficacy of melatonin in insomnia is not very convincing (Buscemi et al. 2004). Over-the-counter melatonin is not FDA approved for insomnia and isn't regulated. Doctors sometimes use melatonin to treat body-clock problems such as jet lag, although this practice hasn't been sufficiently tested.

substance use as a potential safety behavior

Using caffeine, alcohol, cigarettes, and sleep medications (whether prescribed, herbal, or over-the-counter) may actually be a safety behavior for you and, thus, a sleep-interfering factor.

Remember, a safety behavior is something you do to try to avoid potentially unpleasant experiences, such as being awake at night or feeling fatigued during the day. For example, you may smoke a cigarette to stave off feelings of anxiety before bedtime, drink alcohol to help you fall asleep more quickly, consume caffeine to avoid feeling tired, or take a sleeping pill to deal with your fear of not sleeping. These behaviors can reinforce the idea that you're ill equipped to cope, an idea that increases anxiety and interferes with sleep. Some of these behaviors represent high sleep effort, a behavior that we know increases the likelihood that you won't be able to sleep. Using sleep medications because you're anxious about being unable to fall asleep could become a potential sleep-interfering behavior for you.

what about medications for other conditions?

Many people with insomnia also take medications for depression, pain, or anxiety, or for other medical conditions. It would be impossible to review all such medications here. Instead, we make a few brief, general comments about medications taken for depression, anxiety, and pain.

Antidepressant Medications

Antidepressant medications vary in their impact on sleep. Some antidepressant medications may cause or worsen insomnia, others have sedating effects and improve sleep, and others are neutral with respect to sleep. Doctors prescribe some sedating antidepressant medications to patients who have insomnia, even if they're not depressed, although the FDA doesn't indicate using antidepressant medications in the treatment of insomnia. When used to treat sleep, the dose is often lower than the therapeutic antidepressant dose. People vary in the degree to which a given antidepressant affects their sleep. In fact, some medication labels list both sleeplessness and sedation as side effects, so it may be difficult to predict the effect a given antidepressant medication will have on your sleep. If an antidepressant medication disrupts your sleep, you might be tempted to stop using it. However, we emphasize the importance of treating your depression, and recommend discussing emerging side effects with your doctor to determine if it's advisable to change your medication. Sometimes the negative effect of the medication on your sleep is transient. If you're currently depressed, it's most prudent to be treated for depression. Effective treatments for depression include a variety of antidepressant medications and psychotherapies, such as CBT, interpersonal psychotherapy, or short-term dynamic therapy (Chambless et al. 1998). When you have both depression and insomnia, your best strategy is to treat both. In one study, combining the insomnia treatment offered in this book with an antidepressant medication produced a greater improvement in depression than taking an antidepressant medication alone (Manber et al. 2008). The combined treatment also improved sleep to a much greater degree than taking an antidepressant medication alone.

133

Anxiety Medications

Antianxiety medications tend to be either serotonin-related medications (including selective serotonin reuptake inhibitors, or SSRIs, and serotonin-norepinephrine reuptake inhibitors, or SNRIs) or benzodiazepines. Serotonin-related medications are antidepressants and can have a negative effect on sleep in some people. Benzodiazepine antianxiety medications may assist in helping you initially fall asleep, but as with sleeping pills, antianxiety sleep medication can involve tolerance problems; that is, the medications lose their effectiveness, and higher doses are needed to produce the same effect. Stopping this class of medications abruptly may lead to rebound insomnia.

Pain Medications

Because pain can disrupt sleep, it needs to be well managed. A variety of pain medications are used for overall pain management, some of which have an adverse effect on sleep, have no impact on sleep, and may improve sleep. Your doctor may opt to combine pain medications with sleep medications to improve both pain and sleep. Sometimes antidepressant medications are used for pain, and they can have a varying effect on sleep.

---

taking action

1. Continue monitoring your sleep so you can be aware of any changes in your sleep patterns.

2. If the sleep-incompatible behaviors discussed in this chapter apply to you, incorporate our recommendation into worksheet 8.1, "Your Behavioral Plan for Improving Your Sleep." See Gayle's example; she added a goal of not consuming caffeine past 4:00 p.m. and limiting her caffeine consumption to one cup each day. If none of these behaviors applies to you, continue working on past goals you listed on worksheet 5.1, "Your Behavioral Plan for Improving Your Sleep."

3. Listing and addressing safety behaviors using worksheet 8.2, "Changing Safety Behaviors," may also help.

worksheet 8.1 example: Gayle's Behavioral Plan for Improving Her Sleep

Goals for the Week of 5/18–5/24
Check if you met your goal. √

Goals	Monday	Tuesday	Wednesday	Thursday	Friday	Saturday	Sunday
1. I'll leave my bedroom if I'm awake for thirty minutes or more.	√	n/a	√	√	n/a	√	√
2. I'll use my bedroom for sleeping only (no Internet in my bedroom).	√	√	√	√		√	√
3. I won't attempt to nap unless it's necessary for my safety.	√	√	√	√	√	√	√
4. I won't cancel appointments after a poor night's sleep.	√	√	√	√	√	√	√
5. I'll restrict my caffeine consumption to one cup a day and never after 4:00 p.m.	√	√	√	√	√	√	√
6.							
7.							

worksheet 8.1: Your Behavioral Plan for Improving Your Sleep

Goals for the Week of _____ Check if you met your goal. ✓	Monday	Tuesday	Wednesday	Thursday	Friday	Saturday	Sunday
1.							
2.							
3.							
4.							
5.							
6.							
7.							

worksheet 8.2: Changing Safety Behaviors

Safety Behavior	What Message Are You Sending Yourself by Engaging in This Behavior?	What Will You Do to Show That It's Not True?	Result of the Experiment
Example: I take a sleeping pill in the middle of the night when I notice I'm worked up.	It sends a message that I've lost all confidence in my ability to sleep. It also says that I don't think I can cope with feeling worked up.	I'll refrain from taking the pill in the middle of the night and see what happens.	I felt better during the day and less groggy on days I didn't take the pill. Even though it was initially frightening not to take the pill, I noticed that if I took the pill, I tended to fall back to sleep only a few minutes sooner than on nights when I just waited it out.
1.			
2.			
3.			
4.			

summing up

We reviewed several substance-related sleep-incompatible behaviors in this chapter. Sleep-interfering substances include:

- Alcohol

- Cigarettes and other products with nicotine (nicotine patches and nicotine replacement gums)

- Caffeinated beverages and chocolate

Some of these substances interfere with sleep because of direct stimulating effects (for example, caffeine), and others do so because the body's breakdown of them causes a sleep-disruptive rebound (for example, alcohol).

People sometimes use substances as a safety behavior to avoid negative feelings from lying awake in bed for a long time and feeling tired the next day. Safety behaviors reaffirm the idea that you can't cope, and erode your confidence in your sleep ability, both of which make you anxious and interfere with sleep.

General Guidelines

- Take sleep medications only as prescribed.

- If you take sleep medications nightly, it's best to take them at bedtime rather than first trying to sleep without them.

- Avoid alcohol consumption within a few hours of bedtime, and limit consumption to one to two drinks.

- Quit smoking or using other nicotine products.

- Limit caffeine consumption to less than 250 milligrams of caffeine each day (an average mug of coffee has just over half this amount).

- Never consume caffeine within four to six hours of your bedtime.

CHAPTER 9

when things get in the way of treatment

Now that we've covered the essentials of the treatment, let's consider some potential barriers to change and ways to overcome them. In addition we'll discuss implementing this book's strategies in the face of the unique challenges sometimes associated with suffering from another condition along with insomnia. Finally, we'll provide some solutions to these potential challenges.

what do you see as barriers to treatment?

Our clinical experience has taught us that treatments are most effective when we explore and understand individual barriers to following our various recommendations. We encourage you to identify and develop plans to address the barriers that make it difficult to follow our recommendations. The first step is to identify the ones that might be particularly challenging for you.

1. How likely are you to follow each of these recommendations?

Core Strategies	Not at all likely	Slight chance	Fairly likely	Very likely
Leave the room when you're unable to sleep.	0	1	2	3
Avoid wakeful activities in the bedroom.	0	1	2	3
Decrease safety behaviors.	0	1	2	3
Avoid *trying* to sleep.	0	1	2	3
Maintain a regular rise time.	0	1	2	3
Challenge thoughts that disrupt sleep.	0	1	2	3
Restrict your time in bed to match the current amount of sleep your body produces.	0	1	2	3

2. For the recommendations you rated 0 or 1, what do you think might get in the way of following these recommendations?

Recommendation	Barrier to Making a Change
Example: Avoid wakeful activities in bed.	My spouse likes to watch television in bed and will get upset if I suggest we turn it off.
1.	
2.	
3.	
4.	
5.	

3. Can you come up with possible solutions to these barriers?

Recommendation	Barrier to Change	Possible Solution
Example: Avoid wakeful activities in bed.	My spouse likes to watch television in bed and will get upset if I suggest we turn it off.	Maybe my spouse would be open to watching TV in the living room. My spouse would like me to sleep better; maybe if I explain why, he would understand.
1.		
2.		
3.		
4.		
5.		

If you're having difficulties identifying solutions to problems that may stand in your way, you might be inspired by some of the following suggestions, offered by fellow insomnia sufferers. As always, if the difficulties persist, you might consider enlisting help from an expert.

possible challenges in implementing change

Next we discuss a few common barriers, emphasizing those that might be most relevant to people who have insomnia along with depression, anxiety, or pain.

Problems with Low Motivation

Feeling unmotivated is a frequent problem for people with depression.

Eric told me (C. E. C.) that my asking him to get out of bed in the morning seemed as likely as his moving an enormous boulder. He saw himself as an immovable object and joked that I should know that it's a scientific principle that an object at rest stays at rest. I agreed that inertia seems to breed inertia and that this was one of the ways in which depression is often perpetuated. The feeling of low energy caused him to rest and cut back on the things he used to do, and the more he was at rest, the more he wanted to stay at rest. However, the boulder doesn't need to feel motivated to be moved; with the right leverage, sometimes a simple push is enough to get a seemingly immovable object to start rolling down a hill. Once rolling, even a boulder gains momentum and eventually moves easily down its path. The initial push can sometimes be accomplished by merely doing something even in the absence of feeling motivated. We frequently rely on feeling motivated to start new projects or do difficult things. I asked Eric how often he felt motivated to do the dishes. He laughed, "Never!" When asked how he managed to avoid doing dishes, Eric replied that he washed dishes even though he didn't feel like doing them. He understood the analogy.

With depression, and some other conditions, you often can't rely on feeling motivated. Sometimes you have to do things even when you don't feel any motivation to do them. Once you're doing the thing you need to do, you'll gain momentum and things may become easier. This process is similar to the proverb: "Fake it till you make it." What if you were to test this theory this week? Pick one of the recommendations to follow over the next week. It might be easiest to start with the one that you're most convinced will be helpful in your situation. Before you start, rate on a scale of 0 to 10 (in which 0 means absolutely no motivation, and 10 means feeling highly motivated to implement the recommendation) how motivated you feel to follow the recommendation. Then, commit and push yourself to do it anyway for a week, just as with doing the dishes or whatever unpleasant activity you do because you have to, regardless of your motivation. We hope that at the end of the week, when you look at your initial rating and what you were able to accomplish, you'll feel encouraged. If you weren't able to accomplish your goal, perhaps you need to identify additional barriers and work through them first. Or maybe you were able to meet the goal only partly, and perfectionism won't allow you to appreciate your progress.

Try starting with more modest expectations. It's also possible that you have an untreated or inadequately treated depressive disorder, in which case you need to talk to your doctor about your depression treatment.

Feeling Overwhelmed by Starting Something New

One of the more difficult challenges you might face is feeling overwhelmed by our recommendations. The first step in addressing this problem is to break each task into smaller, more manageable steps. Consider the following example.

A severe arthritis sufferer, Pat listened to my (C. E. C.) list of recommendations and sighed. When asked what she thought about the treatment, she admitted that she felt overwhelmed by the prospect of making so many changes. I suggested that we focus on two goals and reassess progress in a few weeks to see if she was ready to integrate other components then. We identified two changes that Pat could focus on based on what would likely be most helpful. She was relieved and much more confident that she could make these two changes.

While it's optimal to put all the components together, it's better to implement some recommendations (in steps) than none. If you, like Pat, want to start on a smaller scale, try focusing on the following two recommendations:

- Calculate your time-in-bed prescription and maintain that schedule seven days a week.

- Reserve your bed for sleeping only; that is, get out of bed whenever you can't sleep for a prolonged period.

While implementing all the recommendations yields the most benefit, these two strategies were evaluated as independent treatments and found to be effective (Morin et al. 2006). It's more important to make a change than to perfectly implement all the recommendations. If you continue to encounter difficulties or see no progress, consult a therapist who specializes in treating insomnia. The appendix contains a list of resources, including a website address with a list of treatment providers certified in this type of therapy (www.aasmnet.org).

Difficulty Concentrating

Maybe you have difficulty following this book because your inability to concentrate makes it difficult to remember the paragraph you just read. You may find yourself reading and rereading sections of this book, an experience that can be quite frustrating. If you're having difficulty in this area, one suggestion is to read one paragraph, write down the most important point, and then proceed to reading and summarizing the main point in the next paragraph, and so on. You can also refer to the "Summing Up" section of each chapter, which reiterates the important points of the chapter, and the "Taking Action" section, which sets out the recommended task for the week. It's most important to write down what changes you plan to implement that week. It's far less important to remember every detail. If you have problems concentrating, place ample cues in your environment to help you remember what you need to do. For example, you can leave sticky notes in relevant places as reminders. Perhaps a sticky note on your alarm clock will remind you to stick to your daily rise time, or a sticky note on your computer will remind you to take breaks from sitting at your computer in order to stave off fatigue.

Negative Thoughts

We devoted two chapters to thoughts that can exacerbate insomnia or hinder your following through with the treatment we outlined (chapters 6 and 7). Many people with depression, anxiety, chronic pain, or all of these find it harder to maintain realistic optimism in the face of adversity and challenges. This negative thought process may interfere with efforts to implement the treatment. Thoughts like "This will never work" or "I'll never be able to do this" tend to erode confidence in your ability to accomplish challenging tasks. The good news is that this book's strategies for overcoming insomnia will likely work whether or not you believe in them. It's not a requirement to believe that they'll work. This means that the only requirement is that you give them a try. If you're asking yourself, "What's the point of trying?" consider answering, "I'll give it an honest try for the next month and see if it works for me." Since you've put energy into getting this book and reading this far, it seems that you're motivated to resolve your sleep problem. If this book doesn't help you, you'll know within a month, so why not try something that may work rather than do what you've been doing (which we know isn't working)? If you're having pessimistic thoughts but decide, nonetheless, to try the program for a month, it's important to pay attention to progress, however small. You'll need to open your field of vision and see the two parts of a half-filled glass, the empty space and the full space. If you fail to notice progress, you'll become discouraged and find the program even more difficult to follow. Ron's example illustrates this point.

Suffering with chronic intractable foot pain, Ron took one to two hours to fall asleep, was awake in the middle of the night for two to three hours, and felt very tired during the day. He committed to restricting his time in bed. Two weeks later, when I (C. E. C.) asked him how he was progressing, he replied, "Not good." I reviewed his sleep log and found that he now reported falling asleep within a half hour and being up in the middle of the night for thirty to forty-five minutes, but his fatigue ratings had improved only slightly. I was struck by the discrepancy between the remarkable improvement in his sleep and his failure to see his progress. It turned out that he was focused on the half-empty glass ("I still feel fatigued during the day"), while ignoring the half-full glass (his sleep had improved). Encouraged by our discussion of his progress and its limits, Ron continued with the program until he was sleeping seven and a half hours and his sleep was interrupted by only one brief trip to the bathroom, yet he continued to feel fatigued during the day. We rejoiced in his progress (the half-full glass). This time, it was equally important to pay attention to his fatigue (the half-empty glass). He consulted his physician, who discovered that Ron had iron deficiency, which was successfully treated, allowing his energy levels to return to normal.

Sometimes thoughts that cause negative feelings make it difficult to fall asleep or stay asleep, or make it more difficult to cope on days after a poor night's sleep. In these cases, it's important to leave the bedroom and return only when you feel you're able to sleep, as we discussed in chapter 6. Other helpful strategies in such cases are to maintain a wind-down period before bedtime and use worksheet 7.1, "Thought Worksheet." The analogy of the scratched CD that gets stuck in a groove fits here too. Sometimes negative thoughts can become almost automatic. People with depression, anxiety, and chronic pain sometimes get into a thought rut, wherein their thinking becomes consistently negative. When you catch yourself having troublesome negative thoughts, we recommend completing a thought worksheet, which invites you to critically evaluate whether the thought is fully accurate or helpful. With time you'll learn to do it in your head, interrupting the automatic negative process and helping yourself get unstuck. This is one of the techniques used in cognitive behavioral therapy for a variety of conditions, including depressive and anxiety disorders, and chronic-pain management. The content of the thoughts may be different for depression, anxiety, and insomnia disorders, but the strategy is the same for addressing the negative thoughts. For example, the negative thoughts in insomnia may focus on the cause of insomnia and worry about the consequences of sleeping poorly. People with depression tend to experience thought content characterized by self-criticism. The thought content for people with anxiety disorders tends to focus on fears and worries. Last, people with chronic pain tend to think worry-related thoughts about injury and the catastrophic implications of their pain for future functioning. If your thinking is characterized by self-criticism or perfectionism, you're more likely to be self-punitive when you encounter problems with following this insomnia treatment. Self-criticism is rarely an effective motivational strategy for human beings. Ask yourself, "If someone I loved were following a treatment, would I declare that person worthless for not following it perfectly? The answer is undoubtedly no, because we all want to support our loved ones, and we know that it's more difficult for us to achieve our goals when we feel low. Treat yourself as patiently and supportively as you would treat someone you loved who was embarking on a project such as this. Following is an example of a thought worksheet that's relevant to negative self-talk.

worksheet 9.1 example: Thought Worksheet

Situation	Mood	Distressing Thoughts or Images	Evidence the Most Distressing Thought Is True	Evidence the Most Distressing Thought May Not Be True	Balanced Alternative Thoughts	Current Mood Rating
Describe the situation in which the distressing thought arose.	*Describe mood in one word and rate its intensity (0–100%)*	*Write any thoughts or images going through your mind. Does this thought activate fears about your well-being or how others may view you?*	*Circle the most distressing thought in the previous column. Write factual evidence for this distressing thought. Stay away from evidence that's not factual; for example, a thought that "feels" true is not factually true.*	*Write evidence that doesn't support this thought; have you had experiences that show that this thought isn't true 100% of the time?*	*Write a thought that better summarizes the evidence for the distressing thought.*	*Copy your feelings from column 2. Rerate the intensity of the feelings.*
Slept in again today.	Angry with self (90%)	(I'm useless.)	I haven't been able to follow the rise-time recommendation at all.	I followed the recommendation three times during the first week.	Although I've had trouble following one of the recommendations this week, this doesn't mean I'm useless.	Angry with self (40%)
	Depressed (80%)	I can't even get out of bed.	I napped one day last week.	I've followed other recommendations this week.	I'll feel more motivated if I refrain from harsh self-criticism.	Depressed (20%)
		Got an image of my dad yelling at me when I was a little kid for screwing up.	It seems that whenever I put my mind to something, I can only stick to it for a week.	My daughter doesn't think I'm useless. I do a pretty good job of taking care of her on my own.		
		Why can't I follow these simple rules?		Not following a treatment probably doesn't mean that I'm completely useless.		
		I'll always have sleep problems.		I wouldn't think my friend was useless if he had trouble getting out of bed in the morning.		

146

When You Don't Want to Get Out of Bed

When life appears to offer little incentive to leave the bedroom, it's difficult to adhere to a fixed wake time and motivate yourself to get out of bed. When you stay in bed, you have fewer opportunities to experience the positive aspects of life. After all, how many truly interesting things happen when you're always in bed? Staying in bed is particularly problematic when a person is already depressed, because it reduces access to pleasurable activities and therefore confirms a worldview that life has no potential for enjoyment. Staying in bed can also perpetuate anxious feelings and thoughts, because the more you avoid leaving your home, the fewer opportunities you have to face your fears and prove them wrong. If life outside of your home produces fears of injury, social interaction, exposure to germs, having a panic attack, or whatever the fear may be, then you can develop a tendency to avoid leaving your home, which further perpetuates the fears. Similarly, it's tempting to stay in bed when you're in pain out of fear of having more pain or getting injured. This might be a good strategy immediately after an injury or surgery, but inactivity is not a good long-term strategy to deal with chronic pain because it weakens the muscles and makes you prone to more injuries.

Difficulty getting out of bed in the morning can also stem from a delay in your body clock. If you have a delayed body clock, you might try to wake up before your clock sends sufficiently strong alerting signals. If you let yourself sleep in when you have no obligations (for example, on the weekend), you're weakening the signal from your body clock because the body clock relies on regular wake time and light exposure. In each of these scenarios, being resistant to getting up and staying indoors in the morning rather than getting sunlight will significantly interfere with your progress.

There are two approaches to troubleshooting these issues. One is the "fake it till you make it" method mentioned earlier; that is, follow the guideline even when you're not motivated to do it. Although motivation enhances everything we do, waiting until you're motivated might not be a good strategy, because in the meanwhile, staying in bed will likely make you feel worse and further weaken your body clock. One trick to getting out of bed without relying on motivation is to swing your legs onto the floor as soon as you hear the alarm, because it's difficult to fall back to sleep in this position. Another trick is to set a loud alarm on a clock placed across the room from your bed so that you have to get out of bed to turn it off. Enlisting others to wake you is effective for some people. Make it a cardinal rule that getting back into bed is *forbidden* and that you won't break this rule under any circumstances. If you push yourself to get out of bed despite feeling unmotivated, be sure to pay attention to any successes or improvements in sleep quality, however small, which will help you to continue pressing on with the program and ultimately will help you sleep much better.

Another strategy is to make it more rewarding to get out of bed and the bedroom. Identify activities you enjoy and, if possible, schedule them for shortly after you wake up. Setting yourself up for success will necessitate some advance thinking about these issues; worksheet 9.2, "Enjoying Your Morning," (later in this chapter) may help in this regard. Almost universally, people find that it feels better to get out of bed and leave the bedroom, even if they initially didn't feel like it. Failing to leave the bedroom often leads to boredom (because there's not much to do in the bedroom), a sense of purposelessness (feeling as if you haven't accomplished anything or that your life is empty), or anxiety (about the things you need to do that didn't get done because you were in bed). But don't take our word for it; set up an experiment to test whether this is true. First take a week to monitor how you feel when you give in to the temptation to stay in bed. Then for the next week, monitor how you feel when you force yourself to leave the bed even when you don't feel like it. We think you'll be pleasantly surprised.

When Fear of Panic Attacks Keeps You Awake

Some people have panic attacks in their sleep. They awaken in sudden fear with a number of symptoms, such as heart palpitations, rapid breathing, and a choking sensation. Called *nocturnal panic*, this condition can be very upsetting, potentially leading to a fear of sleep. Nocturnal panic may begin as a misfiring of the *fight-or-flight* system in response to small changes in breathing or muscle activity during sleep. The fight-or-flight reaction involves activation of several body systems (for instance, faster heart rate and respiration, sweating, clammy hands) in preparation to face a potential threat. In nocturnal panic, the misfiring occurs in the absence of a real threat or actual danger. People with nocturnal panic appear to be particularly sensitive, albeit without awareness, to small and normal physical changes that occur during the transition between sleep stages. Researchers believe that after waking up in the middle of the night, the person interprets the panic symptoms as a sign that something is terribly wrong, which further escalates the fear symptoms, potentially producing a full-blown panic attack (Craske and Freed 1995). For example, a common physical symptom of nocturnal panic is feeling out of breath upon awakening, a symptom often interpreted as a sign of possible suffocation, which leads to intense fear.

We won't address treatment of nocturnal panic attacks here, because it deserves a separate book. But briefly, treatment of panic disorder involves learning what panic attacks are, monitoring your attacks and their symptoms so that you can detect their onset early, learning breathing and relaxation techniques to cope with the symptoms, and challenging your beliefs that the physical symptoms of a panic attack are dangerous and intolerable. It's important to recognize that physical sensations during sleep don't pose an actual threat. Normal fluctuations in breathing, heart rate, and muscle activity during sleep can be mistakenly and automatically perceived as danger signs. The appraisal that there's danger when in fact there isn't leads to a response of panic and an intense fear that you'll experience another panic attack. Realizing and reminding yourself that these symptoms are not signs of danger can help you tolerate the panic symptoms and will ironically lessen the severity of panic attacks and make them less likely to reoccur.

If you experience nocturnal panic with choking symptoms, check with your doctor about the possibility that you might also have sleep apnea. As discussed in chapter 2, sleep apnea can involve gasping for breath and the sensation of choking. Some evidence indicates that sleep deprivation may increase panic attacks in some people with panic disorder (Roy-Byrne, Uhde, and Post 1986). If you have panic attacks, you may relax the restriction of your time in bed described in chapter 5 by adding an extra half hour to your time in bed.

Reduced Activities

Many people with insomnia and high job stress look forward to retirement, because they expect their insomnia to resolve with stress reduction. Those whose transition to retirement involves a marked reduction in meaningful activities are often disappointed to discover that their insomnia persists. Besides having reduced stress, they find themselves more socially isolated, doing less, or lacking sufficient stimulation. People with depression, anxiety, and chronic pain also find themselves socially isolated and insufficiently stimulated, though for different reasons, related to their specific problem. Poor sleepers tend to do less on a daily basis, and their daily activities have less regularity (fewer daily routines) than good sleepers (Carney et al. 2006). Why would this contribute to insomnia? Reducing your daily activities weakens the drive for sleep and important cues for the body clock, two factors involved in the regulation of sleep. Low activity levels, social isolation, and insufficient stimulation also contribute to worsening of depressed and anxious mood, and may also worsen pain. When you're already doing less than you used to, you might be daunted by the many treatment-related activities we propose. We recommend increasing your overall activity levels, because we believe that successfully doing so will make it easier to later introduce strategies that felt impossible when you were less active.

If you find that you're understimulated or isolated, or have few regular activities, worksheet 9.1, "Activity Log" (later in this chapter), might help. Start by monitoring your current activities and pay attention to your mood in relation to your level of engagement in activities. Pay attention even to small variations in activity levels and mood. We hope you'll find that the more you do, the better you'll feel, even though initially you may not feel like doing anything. Then *gradually* increase your daily activities. Ideally, also introduce and maintain some regularity in your new schedule, a strategy called *behavioral activation*. Research shows that this strategy improves depressed mood and fatigue, and increases motivation (Gortner et al. 1998). Research also shows that those suffering from chronic fatigue and pain conditions also benefit from increasing activities, as long as the increase is gradual and the activities are paced (allowing time to rest, but not nap, between activities), an approach that improves mood and stamina, and reduces pain (Fulcher and White 1997).

If you find that fears of reinjury or exposure to anxiety-provoking situations prevent you from doing activities you listed in worksheet 9.1, "Activity Log," chances are you're engaging in safety behaviors. We discussed in chapter 7 how safety behaviors (things you do to avoid a feared outcome) actually perpetuate insomnia problems. The same holds true for anxiety and chronic pain. If you avoid doing things to keep from experiencing anxiety or reinjury, your fear will only grow, which highlights the importance of resisting safety behaviors. Worksheet 7.2, "Changing Safety Behaviors," may help in this regard. Remind yourself of the negative consequences of a safety behavior, for example, that it increases the likelihood of perpetuating the problem. As you increase your activities, gain momentum, and feel better, you may feel ready to start with our suggested activities for improving your insomnia.

When Nightmares or "Bad Dreams" Disturb Your Sleep

In some cases, having recurrent bad dreams or nightmares leads to fear of going to sleep and of having insomnia. Nightmares are common in people who've experienced a trauma, including those diagnosed with PTSD. If this applies to you, you would likely benefit from trauma-focused treatment. We recommend that you also treat your insomnia, because up to half of people treated for PTSD who recover may continue to have significant insomnia (Zayfert and DeViva 2004). If nightmares remain an issue after treatment, or if your nightmares are unrelated to trauma, consider the strategy described next.

The next strategy is most applicable when you can identify recurring themes in your nightmares. It's not uncommon to initially believe that nightmares are random, but as you reflect on their content and applicability to your daytime events, you'll likely identify a few themes. You might notice that the general theme of your dream or nightmare includes some of your daytime experiences or concerns. The strategy for reducing the frequency and intensity of unwanted dreams and nightmares is called *dream rehearsal* or *imagery rehearsal*. Write down the content of the dream or nightmare currently bothering you. If you've identified several themes, choose one to start with. Be sure to include as much detail as possible. Then rewrite the story of the dream by changing it so that it's no longer a nightmare. For most people this means that they change the ending of the dream. Once you're satisfied with this new dream, take at least twenty minutes to imagine the dream as richly and vividly as possible. In your mind's eye, imagine all the details of this new, less scary dream. Practicing this new dream will make it more likely that the old dream will occur less frequently, and generally, when this old dream recurs, it's usually far less disturbing and thus far less likely to cause insomnia. Some people report that this practice helps them alter the story of their dreams as they occur, preventing them from becoming nightmares. Keep up with this practice until you see the results you want, bearing in mind that it may take practice to master the technique. Completing worksheet 9.3, "Nightmare Log," at the end of this chapter may help you track your progress. Though remembering a bad dream isn't pleasant, as you reexperience it, you may also find that you become more detached from the bad dream, to the point where it becomes a story or just a dream. As you step in and alter your dreams, you feel less helpless and eventually master your nightmare experiences. We caution against using this technique with trauma-related dreams without the help of a therapist.

worksheet 9.1: Activity Log Week of _____

TIME	MON Activity/Mood (0–100%)	TUE Activity/Mood (0–100%)	WED Activity/Mood (0–100%)	THUR Activity/Mood (0–100%)	FRI Activity/Mood (0–100%)	SAT Activity/Mood (0–100%)	SUN Activity/Mood (0–100%)
Example: 8:00 a.m.	Drove kids to school (80% happy)	Slept in (30% depressed)	Canceled lunch with friends (60% anxious)	Drove kids to school (60% happy)	Watched TV (90% tired)	Watched TV (90% tired)	Went to church (40% nervous)
7:00 a.m.							
8:00 a.m.							
9:00 a.m.							
10:00 a.m.							
11:00 a.m.							
noon							
1:00 p.m.							
2:00 p.m.							
3:00 p.m.							
4:00 p.m.							
5:00 p.m.							
6:00 p.m.							
7:00 p.m.							
8:00 p.m.							
9:00 p.m.							
10:00 p.m.							
11:00 p.m.							
midnight							

Relationship Issues

You might be concerned that some of your changes in sleep habits may interfere with your bed partner's sleep or that the changes will be met with resistance from your partner. However you may be surprised to find that your partner is more concerned with helping you sleep better than any minor inconvenience to his or her own sleep. Also, your partner might sleep very soundly and not even notice when you get out of bed because you can't sleep. Chances are that your partner will readily fall back to sleep if awaked by you, assuming that your partner doesn't also suffer from insomnia. If your partner does have insomnia, the two of you may benefit from following the treatment together. We therefore encourage you to discuss your concerns with your partner. If your partner isn't initially supportive, some negotiation may be necessary. The first step is to communicate clearly what you would like and why you're asking. Identify the components of the program in which you don't feel supported, and clearly explain the rationale for each of them. If your partner isn't convinced, you'll need to find a compromise.

Jeanne was successful in following many of the treatment recommendations, but when she asked her husband to turn off the television in their bedroom, he was unwilling. She explained why she needed the television to be turned off while she was in bed, but her husband complained that it was a habit that he was unwilling to break. Her husband suggested that he set the TV timer for thirty minutes so it wouldn't be on all night. Although this was a step in the right direction, Jeanne was concerned that a half hour of wakeful activity in bed might not allow her to get the maximal benefit from the treatment. Jeanne suggested that he set the timer for thirty minutes but that she delay her bedtime by the same amount of time so she would get into bed just as the television was about to turn off. Her husband agreed to this compromise.

For best results when negotiating a solution, follow these five guidelines:

- Be very clear about what you're requesting.

- Communicate your request directly and with care.

- Stay focused on what you want to communicate (don't allow yourself to be led away from the issue) and refocus the conversation if it strays.

- Understand and respect your partner's needs.

- Be willing to tolerate a negative reaction.

Do I Have to Do This for the Rest of My Life?

A commonly asked question is, "Must I follow this program for the rest of my life?" a prospect you may find daunting. Indeed, you may find it difficult to follow a schedule seven days a week, limit your time in bed, get out of bed when you can't sleep, refrain from napping, or limit caffeine and alcohol consumption. You might know people who sleep perfectly well but don't follow all, or even some, of these guidelines. However, these recommendations are known to help people with insomnia sleep better. When you no longer have insomnia, you may not need to follow these guidelines so strictly. In fact we hope you'll sleep so well that you'll no longer give sleep much thought. When you're sleeping well and trust that the improvement is here to stay, you can experiment with relaxing some of the sleep guidelines. It may be best to try relaxing one component at a time for a few weeks and then start relaxing another component. This stepwise method will allow you to pinpoint and resume using only those guidelines that are particularly important for you. For example, in chapter 5 we provided guidelines for systematically increasing your time spent in bed when your sleep is solid but you still feel tired during the day. In contrast, when you feel that your sleep is getting worse, it's probably time to bring back the guideline for restricting your time in bed. Some people may have to follow the guidelines indefinitely because of a more-fragile sleep system, but generally, most people will be able to relax some of these guidelines and continue to sleep well. It's important to note, however, that the sleep guidelines provided in this book are designed to optimize your sleep and help prevent future sleep problems. So you may opt to maintain these healthy sleep behaviors permanently, as long as doing so doesn't compromise your quality of life.

---

taking action

If you're having any difficulty implementing this book's strategies, complete whatever worksheets in this chapter apply to you. For example, if you need to systematically increase your activities, use worksheet 9.1, "Activity Log." If getting out of bed in the morning has been a challenge, use worksheet 9.2, "Enjoying Your Morning." Similarly, if bad dreams are interfering with your sleep, you may opt to use worksheet 9.3, "Nightmare Log," to guide your "re-scripting" of troublesome dreams.

worksheet 9.2: Enjoying Your Morning

Are you having trouble getting out of bed in the morning? If so, it may help to identify what you see as the barrier. For example:

- Don't want to face the day?

- Too comfy in bed?

- Hate mornings?

- Not a morning person?

- Believe you have nothing to look forward to?

- Are you convinced that you may be able to fall asleep again?

These are all common problems. Coming up with a good solution will improve your ability to follow through with getting out of bed in the morning. Following are some solutions that our clients have found helpful. The best solution is one that comes from you, so we hope this list inspires you to come up with your own solution. Many of these solutions involve scheduling something pleasurable in the morning.

Possible Solutions:

- Go directly into the shower to increase alertness.

- Make yourself a special breakfast.

- Treat yourself by buying or brewing your favorite coffee or tea.

- Go out for breakfast; think about making it a weekly ritual.

- Take your dog for a walk, or if you don't have a dog, go by yourself. Fresh air will make you feel less groggy, and the sun exposure is good for your body clock. (Your dog will thank you!)

- If you enjoy a fancy coffee, treat yourself to an espresso machine or a deluxe coffeemaker to make mornings more special.

- Schedule a visit with a friend.

- Put the comforter or quilt from your bed in your favorite chair in the house. Moving from a cozy bed to a comfy chair will ease the transition.

- Remind yourself that if you get any more sleep, it will be light sleep at best, because for most of us, extra sleep in the morning tends to be light.

- _____

_____

worksheet 9.3: Nightmare Log

Day of the Week: (When you woke from a nightmare)	Example: Monday						
Calendar Date:	3/25/05						
I had ____ total nightmares last night.	4						
Rate the intensity of each nightmare on a 10-point scale, in which 1 = not at all disturbing, 5 = moderately disturbing, and 10 = extremely disturbing.							
Nightmare 1	2						
Nightmare 2	5						
Nightmare 3	1						
Nightmare 4	8						
Nightmare 5							
Nightmare 6							
Sum of Nightmare Ratings:	16						
I was awakened from sleep by nightmares _____ times.	2						
My awakenings due to nightmares lasted _____ minutes (list each awakening separately).	20 min. 45 min.						
I would rate the quality of last night's sleep as: 1 = very poor, 2 = poor, 3 = fair, 4 = good, or 5 = excellent.	2						

155

summing up

Things that may get in the way of implementing the treatment outlined in this book include:

- Problems with low motivation

- Feeling overwhelmed by starting something new

- Difficulty concentrating

- Negative thinking

- Not wanting to get out of bed

- Fear of panic attacks at night

- Reduced activities

- Nightmares or "bad dreams"

- Relationship issues

- Believing (and dreading) that you'll have to follow these rules forever

Identifying and troubleshooting these potential problems can help you complete this treatment successfully.

When you can't implement components of this treatment, you might benefit from consulting an insomnia specialist (for resources, see the appendix).

appendix: resources

Many different resources are available for those who have insomnia along with depression, anxiety, and pain. We've compiled a list that may help you find good resources, including some general websites that are aligned with the therapy described in this book (cognitive behavioral therapy). Such sites may provide information and referrals.

Association for Behavioral and Cognitive Therapies (ABCT): ABCT (www.abct.org) is a group dedicated to promoting scientifically supported therapies. At their website, selecting the tab labeled "The Public" gives you access to information about various conditions, including insomnia, depression, anxiety, and pain; information about effective therapies; and a cognitive behavioral therapist locator.

Academy of Cognitive Therapy (ACT): ACT (info@academyofct.org) provides referrals to certified therapists.

American Academy of Cognitive and Behavioral Psychology: AACBP (www.americanacademy ofbehavioralpsychology.org/AABP/FellowDirectory.htm) can provide referrals to board-certified psychologists who specialize in cognitive behavioral therapy.

resources for insomnia

A variety of resources are available for insomnia, including self-help books, support groups, and websites. Following is a list of some popular insomnia resources.

Self-Help Books for Insomnia

Edinger, J. D., and C. E. Carney. 2008. *Overcoming Insomnia: A Cognitive-Behavioral Therapy Approach Workbook.* New York: Oxford University Press.

Glovinsky, P., and A. Spielman. 2006. *The Insomnia Answer: A Personalized Program for Identifying and Overcoming the Three Types of Insomnia.* New York: Perigee Books.

Hauri, P. J., and S. Linde. 1996. *No More Sleepless Nights.* New York: John Wiley and Sons.

Jacobs, G. D. 1998. *Say Good Night to Insomnia: The Six-Week, Drug-Free Program Developed at Harvard Medical School.* New York: Henry Holt and Company.

Morin, C. M. 1996. *Relief from Insomnia: Getting the Sleep of Your Dreams.* New York: Doubleday.

Books About Sleep

Dement, W. C., and Vaughan, C. 2000. *The Promise of Sleep: A Pioneer in Sleep Medicine Explores the Vital Connection Between Health, Happiness, and a Good Night's Sleep.* New York: Dell Publishing.

Lavie, P. 1998. *The Enchanted World of Sleep.* Trans. A. Berris. New Haven, CT: Yale University Press.

Web Resources for Insomnia

National Institutes of Health (NIH): Find the NIH State-of-the-Science Conference Statement on Manifestations and Management of Chronic Insomnia in Adults, June 13 to 15, 2005, at their website consensus.nih.gov/2005/2005InsomniaSOS026html.htm.

National Heart, Lung, and Blood Institute: At their website select "Diseases & Conditions Index" and look for "Insomnia," then select "Sleep Information" and look for "Your Guide to Healthy Sleep" (www.nhlbi.nih.gov/health).

National Sleep Foundation: www.sleepfoundation.org.

Journal of the American Medical Association (JAMA): jama.ama-assn.org/cgi/content /full/295/24/2952.

American Academy of Sleep Medicine: www.aasmnet.org.

Knol on Insomnia: http://knol.google.com/k/rachel-manber/insomnia

self-help books for depression

Bieling, P. J., and M. M. Antony. 2003. *Ending the Depression Cycle: A Step-by-Step Guide for Preventing Relapse.* Oakland, CA: New Harbinger Publications.

Burns, D. D. 1999. *Feeling Good: The New Mood Therapy.* Revised ed. New York: Avon Books.

Greenberger, D., and C. A. Padesky. 1995. *Mind Over Mood: Change How You Feel by Changing the Way You Think.* New York: The Guilford Press.

Strosahl, K. D., and P. J. Robinson. 2008. *The Mindfulness and Acceptance Workbook for Depression: Using Acceptance and Commitment Therapy to Move Through Depression and Create a Life Worth Living.* Oakland, CA: New Harbinger Publications.

Web Resources for Depression

Depression and Bipolar Support Alliance: www.dbsalliance.org.

National Alliance on Mental Illness: www.nami.org.

Mood Disorders Society of Canada: www.mooddisorderscanada.ca.

self-help books for anxiety

Antony, M. M., and R. E. McCabe. 2004. *10 Simple Solutions to Panic: How to Overcome Panic Attacks, Calm Physical Symptoms, and Reclaim Your Life.* Oakland, CA: New Harbinger Publications.

Antony, M. M., and R. P. Swinson. 2008. *The Shyness and Social Anxiety Workbook: Proven Step-by-Step Techniques for Overcoming Your Fear.* 2nd ed. Oakland, CA: New Harbinger Publications.

—————. 2009. *When Perfect Isn't Good Enough: Strategies for Coping with Perfectionism.* 2nd ed. Oakland, CA: New Harbinger Publications.

Asmundson, G. J. G., and S. Taylor. 2005. *It's Not All in Your Head: How Worrying About Your Health Could Be Making You Sick—And What You Can Do About It.* New York: The Guilford Press.

Barlow, D. H., and M. G. Craske. 2007. *Mastery of Your Anxiety and Panic* Workbook. 4th ed. New York: Oxford University Press.

Bourne, E. J. 2005. *The Anxiety and Phobia Workbook.* 4th ed. Oakland, CA: New Harbinger Publications.

Bourne, E. J., and L. Garano. 2003. *Coping with Anxiety: 10 Simple Ways to Relieve Anxiety, Fear, and Worry.* Oakland, CA: New Harbinger Publications.

Gyoerkoe, K. L., and P. S. Wiegartz. 2006. *10 Simple Solutions to Worry: How to Calm Your Mind, Relax Your Body, and Reclaim Your Life.* Oakland, CA: New Harbinger Publications.

Hope, D. A., R. G. Heimberg, H. R. Juster, and C. L. Turk. 2000. *Managing Social Anxiety: A Cognitive-Behavioral Therapy Approach—Client Workbook.* New York: Oxford University Press.

Kabat-Zinn, J. 1990. *Full Catastrophe Living: Using the Wisdom of Your Body and Mind to Face Stress, Pain, and Illness.* New York: Dell Publishing.

Purdon, C., and D. A. Clark. 2005. *Overcoming Obsessive Thoughts: How to Gain Control of Your OCD.* Oakland, CA: New Harbinger Publications.

Rothbaum, B. O., E. B. Foa, and E. A. Hembree. 2007. *Reclaiming Your Life from a Traumatic Experience: Workbook.* New York: Oxford University Press.

Web Resources for Anxiety

Anxiety Disorders Association of America: www.adaa.org.

Anxiety Disorders Association of Canada: www.anxietycanada.ca.

NIMH Anxiety Disorders brochure: www.nimh.nih.gov/health/publications/anxiety-disorders/summary.shtml.

Anxieties.com: www.anxieties.com.

Freedom From Fear: www.freedomfromfear.org.

---

self-help books for chronic pain

Currie, S., and K. Wilson. 2002. *60 Second Sleep-Ease: Quick Tips to Get a Good Night's Rest.* Far Hills, NJ: New Horizon Press.

Friedberg, F. 2006. *Fibromyalgia and Chronic Fatigue Syndrome: 7 Proven Steps to Less Pain and More Energy.* Oakland, CA: New Harbinger Publications.

Gardner-Nix, J. 2009. *The Mindfulness Solution to Pain: Step-by-Step Techniques for Chronic Pain Management.* Oakland, CA: New Harbinger Publications.

Lewandowski, M. J. 2006. *The Chronic Pain Care Workbook: A Self-Treatment Approach to Pain Relief Using the Behavioral Assessment of Pain Questionnaire.* Oakland, CA: New Harbinger Publications.

Web Resources for Chronic Pain

Pain Connection: www.painconnection.org.

American Pain Foundation: www.painfoundation.org.

American Chronic Pain Association: www.theacpa.org.

National Institute of Arthritis and Musculoskeletal and Skin Diseases: www.niams.nih.gov.

Exercise: A Guide from the National Institute on Aging: weboflife.nasa.gov/exercise andaging/toc.html.

American Pain Society: www.ampainsoc.org.

International Association for the Study of Pain: www.iasp-pain.org.

American College of Rheumatology: www.rheumatology.org.

The American Fibromyalgia Syndrome Association: www.afsafund.org.

resources for quitting smoking

Many effective treatments are available to help you stop smoking, and your family doctor may be a good resource for additional info or for finding a local support group. Here's an online support group to try: www.quitsmokingsupport.com. Following is a helpful publication.

Antonuccio, D. O. 1992. *Butt Out: The Smoker's Book: A Compassionate Guide to Helping Yourself Quit Smoking, With or Without a Partner.* Saratoga, CA: R & E Publishing.

resources for communicating needs in a relationship

Relationship issues can frequently play a role in your ability to stick to this treatment. In some cases relationship conflict creates stress and interferes with sleep. Sometimes a partner's habits (for example, leaving the television on throughout the night) or medical condition (such as snoring or sleep apnea) may directly affect your sleep. In other cases, your bed partner may object to the parts of this treatment that could potentially affect his or her sleep. Following are some helpful publications, but also consider enlisting the help of a therapist who has an expertise in relationship issues.

Christensen, A., and N. S. Jacobson. 2000. *Reconcilable Differences.* New York: The Guilford Press.

Davis, M., K. Paleg, and P. Fanning. 2004. *The Messages Workbook: Powerful Strategies for Effective Communication at Work and Home.* Oakland, CA: New Harbinger Publications.

Paterson, R. J. 2000. *The Assertiveness Workbook: How to Express Your Ideas and Stand Up for Yourself at Work and in Relationships.* Oakland, CA: New Harbinger Publications.

references

Adamson, J., and J. A. Burdick. 1973. Sleep of dry alcoholics. *Archives of General Psychiatry* 28 (1):146–49.

Agargün, M. Y., H. Kara, and M. Solmaz. 1997. Sleep disturbances and suicidal behavior in patients with major depression. *Journal of Clinical Psychiatry* 58 (6):249–51.

American Psychiatric Association (APA). 2000. Diagnostic and Statistical Manual of Mental Disorders, 4th ed., text rev. (DSM-IV-TR). Washington, DC: American Psychiatric Association.

Aschoff, J., and R. Wever. 1981. The circadian system of man. In *Biological rhythms: Handbook of behavioral neurobiology*, ed. J. Aschoff, 311–31. New York: Plenum Press.

Benloucif, S., L. Orbeta, R. Ortiz, I. Janssen, S. I. Finkel, J. Bleiberg, and P. C. Zee. 2004. Morning or evening activity improves neuropsychological performance and subjective sleep quality in older adults. *Sleep* 27 (8):1542–51.

Bonnet, M. B. 2005. Burden of chronic insomnia on the individual. Paper presented at National Institutes of Health State-of-the-Science Conference Statement: Manifestations and Management of Chronic Insomnia in Adults the National Institutes of Health, June 13, Bethesda, MD.

Bonnet, M. H., and D. L. Arand. 1995. 24-hour metabolic rate in insomniacs and matched normal sleepers. *Sleep* 18 (7):581–88.

———. 1996. Insomnia, nocturnal sleep disruption, daytime fatigue: The consequences of a week of insomnia. *Sleep* 19 (6):453–61.

———. 2007. EEG arousal norms by age. *Journal of Clinical Sleep Medicine* 3 (3):271–74.

Bootzin, R. R. 1972. Stimulus control treatment for insomnia. *Proceedings of the 80th Annual Meeting of the American Psychological Association* 7:395–96.

Bootzin, R. R., and P. M. Nicassio. 1978. Behavioral treatments for insomnia. In *Progress in behavior modification*, vol. 6, ed. M. Hersen, R. Eissler, and P. Miller, 1–45. New York: Academic Press.

Borbély, A. A. 1982. A two-process model of sleep regulation. *Human Neurobiology* 1 (3):195–204.

Borkovec, T. D., and B. L. Hennings. 1978. The role of physiological attention-focusing in the relaxation treatment of sleep disturbance, general tension, and specific stress reaction. *Behaviour Research and Therapy* 16 (1):7–19.

Buscemi, N., B. Vandermeer, R. Pandya, N. Hooton, L. Tjosvold, L. Hartling, G. Baker, S. Vohra, and T. Klassen. 2004. Melatonin for treatment of sleep disorders. *Evidence Report: Technology Assessment* 108:1–7.

Buysse, D. J., C. F. Reynolds III, D. J. Kupfer, M. J. Thorpy, E. Bixler, R. Manfredi, A. Kales, A. Vgontzas, E. Stepanski, T. Roth, P. Hauri, and D. Mesiano. 1994. Clinical diagnoses in 216 insomnia patients using the International Classification of Sleep Disorders (ICSD), DSM-IV, and ICD-10 categories: A report from the APA/NIMH DSM-IV Field Trial. *Sleep* 17 (7):630–7.

Buysse, D. J., X. M. Tu, C. R. Cherry, A. E. Begley, J. Kowalski, D. J. Kupfer, and E. Frank. 1999. Pretreatment REM sleep and subjective sleep quality distinguish depressed psychotherapy remitters and nonremitters. *Biological Psychiatry* 45 (2):205–13.

Canals, J., E. Domènech, G. Carbajo, and J. Bladè. 1997. Prevalence of DSM-III-R and ICD-10 psychiatric disorders in a Spanish population of 18-year-olds. *Acta psychiatrica Scaninavica* 96 (4):287–94.

Carney, C. E., and J. D. Edinger. 2006. Identifying critical beliefs about sleep in primary insomnia. *Sleep* 29 (4):444–53.

Carney, C. E., J. D. Edinger, B. Meyer, L. Lindman, and T. Istre. 2006. Daily activities and sleep quality in college students. *Chronobiology International* 23 (3):623–37.

Carney, C. E., Z. V. Segal, J. D. Edinger, and A. D. Krystal. 2007. A comparison of rates of residual insomnia symptoms following pharmacotherapy or cognitive behavioral therapy for major depressive disorder. *Journal of Clinical Psychiatry* 68 (2):254–60.

Carney, C. E., and W. F. Waters. 2006. Effects of a structured problem-solving procedure on pre-sleep cognitive arousal in college students with insomnia. *Behavioral Sleep Medicine* 4 (1):13–28.

Chambless, D. L., M. J. Baker, D. H. Baucom, L. E. Beutler, K. S. Calhoun, P. Crits-Christoph, A. Daiuto, R. DeRubeis, J. Detweiler, D. A. F. Haaga, S. B. Johnson, S. McCurry, K. T. Mueser, K. S. Pope, W. C. Sanderson, V. Shoham, T. Stickle, D. A. Williams, and S. R. Woody. 1998. Update on empirically validated therapies II. *The Clinical Psychologist* 51 (1):3–21.

Clinical Practice Guideline Treating Tobacco Use and Dependence 2008 Update Panel, Liaisons, and Staff. 2008. A clinical practice guideline for treating tobacco use and dependence: 2008 Update—A U.S. Public Health Service report. *American Journal of Preventive Medicine* 35 (2):158–76.

Craske, M. G., and S. Freed. 1995. Expectations about arousal and nocturnal panic. *Journal of Abnormal Psychology* 104 (4):567–75.

Downey, III, R., and M. H. Bonnet. 1992. Training subjective insomniacs to accurately perceive sleep onset. *Sleep* 15 (1):58–63.

Drummond, S. P., J. C. Gillin, and T. L. Smith, and A. DeModena. 1998. The sleep of abstinent pure primary alcoholic patients: Natural course and relationship to relapse. *Alcoholism: Clinical and Experimental Research* 22 (8):1796–1802.

Edinger, J. D., W. K. Wohlgemuth, R. A. Radtke, G. R. Marsh, and R. E. Quillian. 2001. Cognitive behavioral therapy for treatment of chronic primary insomnia: A randomized controlled trial. *Journal of the American Medical Association* 285 (14):1856–64.

España, R. A. and T. E. Scammell. 2004. Sleep neurobiology for the clinician. *Sleep* 27 (4):811–20.

Espie, C. A., N. M. Broomfield, K. M. A. MacMahon, L. M. Macphee, and L. M. Taylor. 2006. The attention-intention-effort pathway in the development of psychophysiologic insomnia: A theoretical review. *Sleep Medicine Reviews* 10 (4):215–45.

Foley, D. J., A. Monjan, S. L. Brown, E. M. Simonsick, R. B. Wallace, and D. G. Blazer. 1995. Sleep complaints among elderly persons: An epidemiologic study of three communities. *Sleep* 18 (6):425–32.

Ford, D. E., and D. B. Kamerow. 1989. Epidemiologic study of sleep disturbances in psychiatric disorders: An opportunity for prevention? *Journal of the American Medical Association* 262 (11):1479–84.

Foster, J. H., and T. J. Peters. 1999. Impaired sleep in alcohol misusers and dependent alcoholics, and the impact upon outcome. *Alcoholism: Clinical and Experimental Research* 23 (6):1044–51.

Fulcher, K. Y., and P. D. White. 1997. Randomized controlled trial of graded exercise in patients with the chronic fatigue syndrome. *British Medical Journal* 314 (7095):1647–52.

Goodman, J. D., C. Brodie, and G. A. Ayida. 1988. Restless leg syndrome in pregnancy. *British Medical Journal* 297 (6656):1101–02.

Gortner, E. T., J. K. Gollan, K. S. Dobson, and N. S. Jacobson. 1998. Cognitive-behavioral treatment for depression: Relapse prevention. *Journal of Consulting and Clinical Psychology* 66 (2):377–84.

Greenblatt, D. J. 1992. Pharmacology of benzodiazepine hypnotics. *Journal of Clinical Psychiatry* 53 (Suppl.):7–13.

Harvey, A. G., and C. Farrell. 2003. The efficacy of a Pennebaker-like writing intervention for poor sleepers. *Behavioral Sleep Medicine* 1 (2):115–23.

Horne, J. A., and O. Östberg. 1976. A self-assessment questionnaire to determine morningness-eveningness in human circadian rhythms. International *Journal of Chronobiology* 4 (2):97–110.

Johnson, C. H. 1990. *An Atlas of Phase Response Curves for Circadian and Circatidal Rhythms.* Nashville, TN: Vanderbilt University Department of Biology.

Levey, A. B., J. A. Aldaz, F. N. Watts, and K. Coyle. 1991. Articulatory suppression and the treatment of insomnia. *Behaviour Research and Therapy* 29 (1):85–89.

Lewinsohn, P. M., and J. Libet. 1972. Pleasant events, activity schedules, and depressions. *Journal of Abnormal Psychology* 79 (3):291–95.

Lichstein, K. L., and T. L. Rosenthal. 1980. Insomniacs' perceptions of cognitive versus somatic determinants of sleep disturbance. *Journal of Abnormal Psychology* 89 (1):105–07.

Manber, R., J. D. Edinger, J. L. Gress, M. G. San Pedro-Salcedo, T. F. Kuo, and T. Kalista. 2008. Cognitive behavioral therapy for insomnia enhances depression outcome in patients with comorbid major depressive disorder and insomnia. *Sleep* 31 (4):489–95.

Matt, G. E., C. Vázquez, and W. K. Campbell. 1992. Mood-congruent recall of affectively toned stimuli: A meta-analytic review. *Clinical Psychology Review* 12 (2):227–55.

Mendelson, W. B., T. Roth, J. Cassella, T. Roehrs, J. K. Walsh, J. H. Woods, D. J. Buysse, and R. E. Meyer. 2004. The treatment of chronic insomnia: Drug indications, chronic use, and abuse liability—Summary of a 2001 New Clinical Drug Evaluation Unit meeting symposium. *Sleep Medicine Reviews* 8 (1):7–17.

Moldofsky, H., P. Scarisbrick, R. England, and H. Smythe. 1975. Musculoskeletal symptoms and non-REM sleep disturbance in patients with "fibrositis syndrome" and healthy subjects. *Psychosomatic Medicine* 37 (4):341–51.

Moore, R. Y. 1994. Organization of the mammalian circadian system. In *Circadian clocks and their adjustment*, ed. J. M. Waterhouse, 88–99. Chichester, West Sussex, UK: John Wiley and Sons.

Morin, C. M. 1993. *Insomnia: Psychological Assessment and Management.* New York: The Guilford Press.

Morin, C. M., R. R. Bootzin, D. J. Buysse, J. D. Edinger, C. A. Espie, and K. L. Lichstein. 2006. Psychological and behavioral treatment of insomnia: Update of the recent evidence (1998–2004). *Sleep* 29 (11):1398–1414.

Morin, C. M., C. Colecchi, J. Stone, R. Sood, and D. Brink. 1999. Behavioral and pharmacological therapies for late-life insomnia: A randomized controlled trial. *Journal of the American Medical Association* 281 (11):991–99.

Morin, C. M., U. Koetter, C. Bastien, J. C. Ware, and V. Wooten. 2005. Valerian-hops combination and diphenhydramine for treating insomnia: A randomized placebo-controlled clinical trial. *Sleep* 28 (11):1465–71.

National Institutes of Health. 2005. State of the Science Conference statement: Manifestations and management of chronic insomnia in adults. *Sleep* 28 (9):1049–57.

National Safety Council. 2001. *Injury Facts.* Itasca, IL: National Safety Council.

Nofzinger, E. A., C. Nissen, A. Germain, D. Moul, M. Hall, J. C. Price, and J. M. Miewald, and D. J. Buysse. 2006. Regional cerebral metabolic correlates of WASO during NREM sleep in insomnia. *Journal of Clinical Sleep Medicine* 2 (3):316–22.

Ohayon, M. M. 2002. Epidemiology of insomnia: What we know and what we still need to learn. *Sleep Medicine Reviews* 6 (2):97–111.

Perlis, M. L., D. E. Giles, D. J. Buysse, X. Tu, and D. J. Kupfer. 1997. Self-reported sleep disturbance as a prodromal symptom in recurrent depression. *Journal of Affective Disorders* 42 (2–3):209–12.

Philips, H. C. 1987. Avoidance behaviour and its role in sustaining chronic pain. *Behaviour Research and Therapy* 25: 273–79.

Rains, J. C. 2008. Chronic headache and potentially modifiable risk factors: Screening and behavioral management of sleep disorders. *Headache* 48 (1):32–39.

Ree, M. J., A. G. Harvey, R. Blake, N. K. Tang, and M. Shawe-Taylor. 2005. Attempts to control unwanted thoughts in the night: Development of the thought control questionnaire-insomnia revised (TCQI-R). *Behaviour Research and Therapy* 43 (8):985–98.

Reynolds III, C. F., and D. J. Kupfer. 1987. Sleep research in affective illness: State of the art circa 1987. *Sleep* 10 (3):199–215.

Roehrs, T., M. Hyde, B. Blaisdell, M. Greenwald, and T. Roth. 2006. Sleep loss and REM sleep loss are hyperalgesic. *Sleep* 29 (2):145–51.

Roehrs, T., and T. Roth. 2001. Sleep, sleepiness, sleep disorders, and alcohol use and abuse. *Sleep Medicine Reviews* 5 (4):287–97.

Roy-Byrne, P. P., T. W. Uhde, and R. M. Post. 1986. Effects of one night's sleep deprivation on mood and behavior in panic disorder: Patients with panic disorder compared with depressed patients and normal controls. *Archives of General Psychiatry* 43 (9):895–99.

Sachs, G. S. 2003. Unmet clinical needs in bipolar disorder. *Journal of Clinical Psychopharmacology* 23 (3, Suppl. 1):2–8.

Salkovskis, P. M. 1991. The importance of behaviour in the maintenance of anxiety and panic: A cognitive account. *Behavioural Psychotherapy* 19:6–19.

Schulz, H., C. Stolz, and J. Müller. 1994. The effect of valerian extract on sleep polygraphy in poor sleepers: A pilot study. *Pharmacopsychiatry* 27 (4):147–51.

Smith, M. T., M. L. Perlis, A. Park, M. S. Smith, J. Pennington, D. E. Giles, and D. J. Buysse. 2002. Comparative meta-analysis of pharmacotherapy and behavior therapy for persistent insomnia. *American Journal of Psychiatry* 159 (1):5–11.

Spielman, A. J., P. Saskin, and M. J. Thorpy. 1987. Treatment of chronic insomnia by restriction of time in bed. *Sleep* 10 (1):45–55.

Sun, E. R., C. A. Chen, G. Ho, C. J. Earley, and R. P. Allen. 1998. Iron and the restless legs syndrome. *Sleep* 21 (4):371–77.

Tang, N. K., and C. Crane. 2006. Suicidality in chronic pain: A review of the prevalence, risk factors, and psychological links. *Psychological Medicine* 36 (5):575–86.

Thase, M. E. 1998. Depression, sleep, and antidepressants. *Journal of Clinical Psychiatry* 59 (Suppl. 4):55–65.

Thase, M. E., A. D. Simons, and C. F. Reynolds III. 1996. Abnormal electroencephalographic sleep profiles in major depression: Association with response to cognitive behavior therapy. *Archives of General Psychiatry* 53 (2):99–108.

U.S. Food and Drug Administration (FDA). 2007. FDA Requests Label Change For All Sleep Disorder Drug Products. www.fda.gov/bbs/topics/NEWS/2007/NEW01587.html. Accessed May 21, 2009.

Van Cauter, E., and F. W. Turek. 1995. Endocrine and other biological rhythms. In *Endocrinology*, 3rd ed., ed. L. J. DeGroot, 2487–548. Philadelphia, PA: WB Saunders.

Verbeek, I., K. Schreuder, and G. Declerck. 1999. Evaluation of short-term nonpharmacological treatment of insomnia in a clinical setting. *Journal of Psychosomatic Research* 47 (4):369–83.

Vitiello, M. V. 1997. Sleep, alcohol, and alcohol abuse. *Addiction Biology* 2:151–58.

Wahlstrom, K. L. 2002. Accommodating the sleep patterns of adolescents within current educational structures: An uncharted path. In *Adolescent sleep patterns: Biological, sociological, and psychological influences*, ed. M. L. Carskadon, 172–197. Cambridge, UK: Cambridge University Press.

Waters, W. F., M. J. Hurry, P. G. Binks, C. E. Carney, L. E. Lajos, K. H. Fuller, B. Betz, J. Johnson, T. Anderson, and J. M. Tucci. 2003. Behavioral and hypnotic treatments for insomnia subtypes. *Behavioral Sleep Medicine* 1 (2):81–101.

Watson, N. F., J. Goldberg, L. Arguelles, and D. Buchwald. 2006. Genetic and environmental influences on insomnia, daytime sleepiness, and obesity in twins. *Sleep* 29 (5):645–49.

Weissman, M. M., S. Greenwald, G. Niño-Murcia, and W. C. Dement. 1997. The morbidity of insomnia uncomplicated by psychiatric disorders. *General Hospital Psychiatry* 19 (4):245–50.

Winkelmann, J., B. Muller-Myhsok, H.-U. Wittchen B. Hock, M. Prager, H. Pfister, A. Strohle, I. Eisensehr, M. Dichgans, T. Gasser, and C. Trenkwalder. 2002. Complex segregation analysis of restless legs syndrome provides evidence for an autosomal dominant mode of inheritance in early age at onset families. *Annals of Neurology* 52 (3):297–302.

Zayfert, C., and J. C. DeViva. 2004. Residual insomnia following cognitive behavioral therapy for PTSD. *Journal of Traumatic Stress* 17 (1):69–73.

Colleen E. Carney, Ph.D., is assistant professor and director of the Sleep and Mood Disorder Program at Ryerson University in Toronto, Canada, and is adjunct professor at Duke University. She is president of the Association for Behavioral and Cognitive Therapies interest group on insomnia and other sleep disorders. Carney was the recipient of the National Sleep Foundation's prestigious Pickwick Fellowship, and her research program is funded by the National Institutes of Health.

Rachel Manber, Ph.D., is professor of psychiatry and behavioral sciences at Stanford University in Palo Alto, CA, where she is also director of the Insomnia and Behavioral Sleep Medicine Program. She has taught many health providers how to use cognitive behavioral therapy for insomnia and is one of the leading authorities on the treatment of comorbid insomnias. Manber's research on depression and insomnia is funded by the National Institute of Mental Health. She is a proponent of empirically supported therapies for those with sleep problems.

Foreword writer **Richard R. Bootzin, Ph.D.,** is professor of psychology and psychiatry at the University of Arizona, director of its sleep research laboratory, and director of the insomnia clinic at University Medical Center.

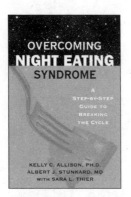
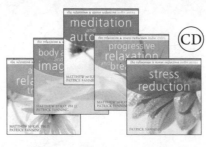
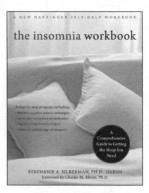
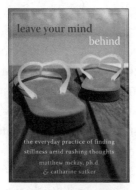
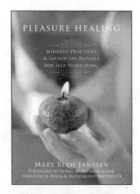
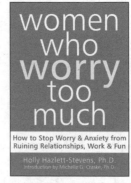